T0136473

Scientific Characters

Scientific Characters

Rhetoric, Politics, and Trust in Breast Cancer Research

Lisa Keränen

The University of Alabama Press
Tuscaloosa

Typeface: Adobe Caslon Pro

∞

The paper on which this book is printed meets the minimum requirements of
American National Standard for Information Sciences-Permanence of Paper for
Printed Library Materials, ANSI Z39.48-1984.

Library of Congress Cataloging-in-Publication Data

Keranen, Lisa.
    Scientific characters : rhetoric, politics, and trust in breast cancer research / Lisa
Keranen.
        p. cm. — (Rhetoric, culture, and social critique)
    Includes bibliographical references and index.
    ISBN 978-0-8173-1704-1 (cloth : alk. paper) — ISBN 978-0-8173-8491-3
(electronic) 1. Breast—Cancer—Research—Moral and ethical aspects. 2.
Scientists—Professional ethics. 3. Scientific surveys. I. Title.
    RC280.B8K48   2010
    362.196′994490072—dc22
                                                                                2009048780

Contents

Acknowledgments

Scientific Characters was neither a stationary nor a solitary endeavor. Portions of this book unfolded on a boat, in high-altitude hippie cafés, in downtown Denver coffeehouses, at seaside resorts, by a lake in Quebec, on frequent airplane trips to Chicago and the East Coast, in my yellow campus office and my green study at home, and on balconies and back porches in Denver, Boulder, New Jersey, Maryland, and Pennsylvania. Three much-abused laptops, numerous creative baristas, and various wireless connections facilitated the entire process. But more than these necessary background materials, the people and institutions that nourished me during the last several years deserve more thanks than I can offer on these pages.

The ideas for this project originated at the University of Pittsburgh, where numerous mentors nurtured my intellectual development and set the stage for the book's completion. Thankfully, this manuscript has grown a great deal from the study that originally inspired it. Nonetheless, John Lyne's insightful critiques of my work and his belief in me and this project buoyed it from conception through revision. John first urged me to pursue the original examination of Fisher's ethos in the Kiva Han coffee shop on Craig Street in Oakland, while Lester Olson, Ted McGuire, Joan Leach, and Pete Simonson boosted the initial project in decisive ways. Other characters from Pitt who shaped me into the thinker and writer I am becoming include Kevin Ayotte, Anand Rao, Lisa Parker, Elizabeth Chaitin, Paul K. J. Han, Henry Krips, Brad Lewis, Gordon Mitchell, Don Egolf, Tim O'Donnell, John Poulakos, David Barnard, Eli Brennan, Omri Ceren, Jukka Keränen, Weiming Yao, Marcus Paroske, and Karen Taylor. Portions of two summers spent shadowing physicians, surgeons, and ethicists at the University of Pittsburgh Medical Center (UPMC) as part of my bioethics training were particularly influential. I also appreciate the unnamed hospital workers, research integrity officers, physicians, lawyers, nurses, and other people affected by federally funded breast cancer research who spoke to me unofficially or off the record and thus cannot be recognized here in any formal way. Most importantly, Lisa Parker and David Sogg gave me shelter at a crucial time. The earliest stages of this book-to-be unfolded in their third-floor study with Zulei the cat for company and David's bassoon echoing through the house.

Friends, colleagues, and students at the University of Colorado (CU) at Boulder have been especially supportive. My summer research assistants over the years—Robert Coombs, Joshua Ehrenreich, Alison Vogelaar, Merrit Dukehart, and Katherine Cruger—assisted with research for this book and many other projects in between. Merrit Dukehart deserves special note for checking my quotations during a flurry of summer activity, and Lauren Archer helped with the bibliography. Meanwhile, the interdisciplinary Rhetoric Workshop, sponsored by CU's Center for the Humanities and the Arts (CHA), provided a testing ground for several chapters in this book, and Karen Tracy, Robert Craig, Jerry Hauser, Rolf Norgaard, John Ackerman, Willard Uncapher, Pete Simonson, the late James McDaniel, and Frank Beer, at various times and in varying degrees, provided first-rate feedback and advice. Throughout, Karen Tracy was my "book buddy"—we traded chapters while she completed *Ordinary Democracy,* and she has since become a cherished friend. At CU–Boulder, my former department chairs, Robert Craig and Michele Jackson, provided structural support while members of the Center for Science and Technology Policy Research (CSTPR) enriched my thinking, especially Roger Pielke and Adam Briggle. Back in the Communication Department, Jane Elvins commented on my French translations and supplied a steady stream of hugs and smiles while Paula Dufour, Katie County, Chris Karman, Josephine Kapatayes, Celia Sinoway, and Julie Blair kept me organized.

In the final stages of this project, I had the great fortune to receive a faculty fellowship from the University of Colorado at Boulder's CHA to begin work on my second book manuscript, a rhetorical history of twentieth-century U.S. biological weapons. During the 2008–2009 academic year, I met every other Wednesday afternoon with a dynamic group of scholars and teachers under the direction of Michael Zimmerman. Although the CHA seminarians helped me envision portions of a different project, they nevertheless provided great cheer and inspiration as I was completing this book.

Friends all along the Front Range of the Rocky Mountains fostered a vibrant intellectual community. Whether we were trying microbrews, skiing, or discussing our foibles over dinner, Greg Dickinson, Brian Ott, April Trees, Larry Frey, Heinrich Schwarz, Christina Foust, Sonja Foss, Barb Walkosz, Brenda J. Allen, Marlia Banning, John Ackerman, Patty Malesh, and Hamilton Bean provided heady conversation and emotional support. I consider myself enriched by each of them. Beyond the Front Range, Judy Segal, Herbert W. Simons, Michael Hyde, J. Robbie Cox, John Angus Campbell, David Depew, the late Joanna Ploeger, James Wynn, Greg Wilson, Deb Dysart-Gale, and Colleen Derkatch were rhetoric of science and medicine mentors, role models, and compatriots.

I thank John Lucaites and staff members at The University of Alabama Press for guiding my manuscript to completion. I further appreciate the sound suggestions of two anonymous reviewers, whose identities (Leah Ceccarelli and Kim Kline) are now unveiled, and my meticulous copyeditor, Jill R. Hughes, all of whom made for a better book. Despite the best efforts of these good people, mine is certainly not a perfect book, nor even the one that I wanted to write; all mistakes of fact or interpretation are mine alone.

On an institutional level, two Andrew Mellon fellowships from the University of Pittsburgh and an award from the Public Address Division of the National Communication Association (NCA) supported my initial study. A summer research stipend and grant for primary documents from the Council on Research and Creative Work (CRCW) at the University of Colorado at Boulder aided the book's conception and writing, while the University of Colorado Denver graciously covered indexing costs. Portions of earlier versions of this work were presented at the New Agendas in Science Communication conference in Austin, Texas, at CU's Center for Science and Technology Policy Research, at annual meetings of the NCA and the Western States Communication Association (WSCA), and at a biennial meeting of the Rhetoric Society of America (RSA). I also shared this project with workshop attendees at the 2007 RSA summer workshop on rhetoric of medicine at Rensselaer Polytechnic Institute, which was led by Sue Wells and Ellen Barton, and presented segments during research presentations at Texas A&M University, the University of Colorado at Boulder, the University of Pittsburgh, and the University of Colorado Denver. Thanks to Richard Street, Robert Craig, Barbara Warnick, and Barbara Walkosz for making those visits possible.

From September 2006 to May 2009, I served as an ethics consultant and member of the clinical ethics committee at Boulder Community Hospital, where a dedicated and courageous group of individuals—Claire Riley, David Kenney, and CeCe Lynch in particular—taught me invaluable lessons about the human face of medicine. I will always be grateful for the ethics committee's poems and meditations, sorrow and laughter, and careful attention to the language used in the art of medicine. I hope to remember what they taught me about the fragility of life, its exquisite pain and shocking beauty, the mysteries of patience and forgiveness, and the gift of *presence* for a long time.

My family, David and Jeanne Belicka, Linda and Ron Bashore, and Laura and Jason Snyder, have been patient while I wrestled with this manuscript and have provided a lifetime of love and support. They all deserve thanks, but my mother, Linda Bashore, especially, and my sister, Laura Belicka Snyder, deserve notice for listening and for their generous proofreading skills. Dad and Jeanne, writing on the boat was a grand if not harrowing experience— thank you for sharing the *Eponines I* and *II.*

My greatest debt is to my darling life partner, Stephen John Hartnett, who unexpectedly arrived bearing sunshine and laughter. He has punctuated my writing with glorious high-altitude hikes, stunning snowshoe adventures, his two radiant children, and unmatched Sicilian dinners. For this—even more than his careful editing, ceaseless conversation, daily care, and all else—he deserves thanks. And so I dedicate this book to him and to my mother, for both share an unwavering luminosity and generosity of spirit.

Acronyms and Abbreviations

AACR	American Association of Cancer Researchers
AEC	Atomic Energy Commission
ACS	American Cancer Society
ASCC	American Society for the Control of Cancer
ASCO	American Society for Clinical Oncology
BCAC	Breast Cancer Advisory Center
BCAM	Breast Cancer Action of Montreal
BCPT	Breast Cancer Prevention Trial
CCNSC	Cancer Chemotherapy National Service Center
CMAJ	*Canadian Medical Association Journal*
HHS	Health and Human Services (some sources use DHHS)
HIV	Human Immunodeficiency Virus
IRB	Institutional Review Board
NAS	National Academy of Science
NABCO	National Alliance of Breast Cancer Organizations
NBCC	National Breast Cancer Coalition
NCI	National Cancer Institute
NEJM	*New England Journal of Medicine*

NIH   National Institutes of Health

NSABP   National Surgical Adjuvant Breast and Bowel Project

NSF   National Science Foundation

NWHN   National Women's Health Network

ORI   Office of Research Integrity

OSI   Office of Scientific Integrity

OSIR   Office of Scientific Integrity Review

OSTP   Office of Science and Technology Policy

PHS   Public Health Service

RCT   Randomized Clinical Trial

Introduction
Trust and Character in Datagate

March 13, 1994, was a disheartening day in the high-stakes world of breast cancer research. The *Chicago Tribune* broke the news with a front-page headline proclaiming "Fraud in Breast Cancer Study: Doctor Lied on Data for Decade."[1] Before this announcement, only a small cadre of medical researchers and government investigators knew that Dr. Roger Poisson, former head of cancer research at Montreal's Saint-Luc Hospital, had previously confessed to falsifying more than one hundred pieces of data used in fourteen U.S.-funded cancer clinical trials.[2] But following the *Tribune's* story, "all hell broke loose," as patients, physicians, politicians, federal investigators, health-care workers, journalists, advocates, and citizens clamored to assess the misconduct's ramifications for North America's premier breast cancer research.[3] They would soon learn that some of the falsifications occurred in Project B-06, the highly influential lumpectomy study that had formed the basis of the National Institutes of Health's (NIH) 1990 consensus statement endorsing breast-conserving lumpectomy with radiation for early-stage breast cancers.[4] Hailed as a major triumph for women's health care, the B-06 project had demonstrated that preserving a breast through lumpectomy and radiation was as effective as removing one or both of those iconic markers of femininity, hence sparing women unnecessary pain and disfigurement.[5] No wonder reports that a researcher had falsified data in a federally funded clinical trial of such magnitude spurred public outcry, enraged women's health advocacy groups, and troubled members of the medical establishment. Harmon Eyre, then deputy vice president of the American Cancer Society (ACS), pronounced the situation "an unmitigated disaster for American women."[6]

As news of the tainted data spread, Dr. Bernard Fisher, then overseer of the B-06 project and a towering giant of cancer research, tumbled from empyrean heights. Never mind that it was Fisher's team who first discovered that Poisson had contributed faulty data to the landmark lumpectomy study, previously published in 1985 and 1989 in the usually unassailable *New England Journal of Medicine*.[7] Never mind that Fisher was not himself accused of falsifying data; the former member of the President's Cancer Advisory Panel was soon forced to resign from a position he had held for more than thirty-five years, was shredded routinely in the mass media, and was called to testify before Congress.[8] Meanwhile, patients fumed, politicians grandstanded, and many stakeholders felt ill-equipped to adjudicate the implications of the flawed data for breast cancer treatment. When the storm began to settle, Fisher was cleared of all wrongdoing, and reanalysis of B-06 data reaffirmed the value of breast conservation.[9] Yet, in the fracturing of rhetorical agency that occurs in such disputes, Fisher's character, like that of other principals in the controversy, was redefined, challenged, and circulated by ensemble—and the process was often muddled and mean. As administrators, politicians, investigators, scientists, patients, activists, journalists, and concerned citizens attempted to make sense of what had happened and to assess the integrity of the now-tarnished research, they asked questions, raised challenges, assigned blame, attributed responsibility, launched and responded to attacks, and ultimately exposed the norms of scientific practice to public scrutiny. Throughout it all, character comprised a sustained topic of debate, showing how scientific knowledge is indelibly shaped by perceptions of the personal temperament, trustworthiness, overall integrity, and transparency of those who produce it.

The controversy that followed widespread publicity of Roger Poisson's data falsification spanned seven years and involved at least two nations, four federal agencies, thirteen academic journals, and eighty-nine collaborative research sites.[10] Its stakeholders included 19 coauthors, 2,163 research participants, the more than 200,000 North American women annually diagnosed with breast cancer and their loved ones, physicians, patients, investigators, health-care workers and advocates, and the broader global citizenry.[11] As the controversy unfolded, the reputations of physician-scientists, clinical trials, breast cancer research, and governmental oversight agencies underwent steady assault; and because of the life-and-death stakes of the outcome of Datagate in terms of breast cancer treatment, patients were inextricably yoked to assessments of scientific character and credibility. Dubbed "NSABP Datagate" by one breast cancer survivor who merged the acronym of the research cooperative that conducted the then tarnished study—the

National Surgical Adjuvant Breast and Bowel Project (NSABP)—with the charge of compromised data, the controversy tapped in to broader anxieties about the relationship between science and its stakeholders, trust and truth, and rhetoric and character in the high-stakes world of medical decision making.[12]

Now that the Datagate imbroglio has faded from public memory, it is time to investigate what the controversy reveals about the intersections of science and publics, rhetoric and character. On its broadest level, this book concerns the roles that rhetoric plays in the dramas of publicly contested biomedical knowledge. More specifically, this book chronicles the relationships between character and knowledge, ethos and episteme, and science and its stakeholders, and reveals the significant force of rhetoric in engendering trust or suspicion in both scientific and public life. Drawing on Datagate as an extended example, I examine how rhetorically constituted characters shaped the controversy's progression, meanings, and outcomes, and consider what happens when scientists, patients, and advocates are called to defend themselves and to contest scientific findings publicly in the high-flying world of biomedical research. In other words, I show how rhetorically constructed characters are imbricated in what Rayna Rapp calls "the immense lumpiness of science," thus detailing how reason and character can be mutually informing.[13] Let me be clear at the outset that I write this book from a position of enormous respect for biomedical science and, in particular, its twentieth-century triumphs; I offer my analysis not as a detraction or denigration of science but as an addition or complement, as a means of revealing the potential challenges and opportunities of the intertwinements of science and character. I demonstrate how various participants in science-based controversies—a term that signifies a tangle of technical and public concerns—make sense of scientific claims based on whom and what they find trustworthy, and how rhetorical processes can foster or undermine trust and thereby shape scientific institutions and practices.[14] In short, I explore what the characters of science-based controversy suggest about the dilemmas of scientific knowledge production in a case that had direct implications for human life and well-being, and I track how various stakeholders wrestled with scientific characters in ways that shaped their perceptions of scientific knowledge, policies, and values.

In the remainder of this introduction, I offer a brief meditation on trust and character in science as a prelude to the central themes of the book, chronicle the contours of the controversy, and conclude with an outline of chapters to come. Throughout, I stress how the primary issue confronting scientists and citizens in Datagate—trust—not only populates the deep background of all scientific endeavors but also is subject to rhetorical processes and investigation. I further consider how the rhetorical nature of trust becomes increasingly important as science assumes greater significance in public policy, decision making, and everyday life. In an era when citizens, politicians, scientists, policymakers, and health-care providers increasingly rely on the scientific testimony of strangers in cases where scientific research affects human life, the need for research integrity is paramount. In an era when scientific findings result from the efforts of hundreds of geographically dispersed investigators, the need for oversight and accountability reigns supreme—both of these conditions require trust in scientists and in the institutions that support scientific research. As philosopher John Hardwig argued, "trust in the testimony of others is necessary to ground much of our knowledge," and "this trust involves trust in the character of the testifiers."[15] In considering the role of trust in Datagate, this book therefore concentrates on character and knowledge as they are rhetorically constituted in the throes of controversy. And as we shall see, in the case of Datagate the stakes involved what many participants believed was nothing short of life and death.

TRUST AND CHARACTER IN SCIENCE

In "Voice as a Summons for Belief," Jesuit-philosopher-turned-media-scholar Walter J. Ong offers a powerful rumination on trust that explicitly links belief and knowledge. Ong maintains that "of the knowledge which individual men have today, almost all is grounded in faith." We know a thing because we believe what we are told. Even the knowledge cultivated by scientists, for Ong, "is almost all grounded in faith, well-founded and rational faith in the reports of their fellow scientists, but faith nevertheless." He explains: "Of the scientific knowledge which any man has, only a tiny fraction has been achieved by his own direct observation. For the rest, he has good reason to believe *that* it is true because, within the limits of their competence, he believes in his fellow scientists reporting on their work or reporting reports of the work of others."[16] Ong thus locates trust at the very core of the scientific enterprise. If others cannot believe, if they cannot have faith in, the words of scientists, then the enterprise loses authority and respect. Ong's observations concerning trust and science highlight a defining dilemma of our time: we are awash in technical information that comes to us via the testimony of strangers. Almost all that we know—what we believe to be true of the heavenly bodies, the earthly realm, and the nature of our own anatomical mysteries—derives from the words of others. Former *New England*

Journal of Medicine editor Arnold S. Relman identified the tangled thicket of trust in science when he wrote, "It seems paradoxical that scientific research, in many ways one of the most questioning and skeptical of human activities, should be dependent on personal trust. But the fact is that without trust the research enterprise could not function."[17] Relman's words illuminate the deep contradiction that the human enterprise most likely to spurn faith in favor of objectivism nonetheless rests firmly on a foundation of belief. The entire scientific project depends on trust in the testimony of strangers, and such trust is cultivated through the use of symbols—that is, through rhetoric, the functional use of language to coordinate social action.

The importance of this tight connection between trust, character, and rhetoric in scientific cases where certainty is impossible and opinions are divided piqued my interest shortly after I moved to Pittsburgh in 1997. One glorious afternoon in early September, I read the *University Times* as I rode the bus home to my Bloomfield neighborhood. An article announcing the university's apology to and financial settlement with one of its distinguished service faculty, Dr. Bernard Fisher, caught my eye. The headline, "Fisher Drops Suit in Exchange for Apology, $2.75 Million," hinted at the years-long saga of miscommunication and misunderstandings that precipitated Fisher's stunning, albeit temporary, fall from grace in a scandal that harmed scientists and breast cancer patients alike.[18] Years later, I set out to investigate what the case could tell us about the roles of trust and character in science-based controversies. To address that question, this book examines how the characters of science-based controversy are cultivated, contested, and maintained; how they are wrestled with in public before they are temporarily set; and how these processes occur within the constraints of intense public and political scrutiny.[19] In short, I argue that the participants of science-based controversies create, modify, and extend rhetorically constituted characters in order to maintain, undermine, or rehabilitate reputations; to challenge or defend scientific norms and knowledge; and to invigorate and resolve disagreements over scientific knowledge, policy, and values. The characterizations that emerge during such controversies thus reveal underlying norms and assumptions about science and its stakeholders, compel particular policy solutions, and divulge some of the key tensions facing scientists and citizens who participate in public science-based controversies. Analysis of the constructed characters of Datagate therefore reveals important lessons for scientists, policymakers, concerned citizens, and scholars of rhetoric and science about the integral role of trust in science and its relation to knowledge and action. In sum, the recurrent characterizations that enlivened Datagate disclose the anxieties and tensions surrounding "big science" in the latter half of the twentieth century and suggest possible lines of rhetorical intervention for scientists and citizens who want to challenge or defend the scientific status quo.

To investigate the mutually influencing roles of trust, rhetoric, and character in Datagate, I develop a theoretical framework grounded in rhetorical studies but enriched by literary theory, science studies, and sociology to show how competing characterizations shape the dynamics and preferred policy solutions of this science-based controversy. This framework compels detailed comparative analyses of the characterizations of the key players in the Datagate controversy across a wide swath of texts, including major newspaper and magazine coverage in the United States and Canada; videotaped television news segments; the professional oncology newsletter the *Cancer Letter;* transcripts of congressional hearings; international medical journal articles, commentary, and case coverage; NSABP historical documents from its founding to the present; and transcribed speeches and interviews. While many of these texts fall within the traditional province of rhetoric and its concerns in the public sphere, others derived from the technical realm but crossed into public discourse as the controversy progressed.[20] Both the scientific/technical and the public sphere texts speak directly to the broader cultural dilemmas concerning the production, interpretation, and negotiation of scientific knowledge.[21] Moreover, these texts testify to a complicated dance of characterization, in which larger battles over science's epistemic authority were rehashed, negotiated, and temporarily settled. Any convincing consideration of science-based controversy, I argue, must account for the vagaries of trust, character, and reputation while illuminating their complicated links to knowledge production.

In interpreting how rhetorically constituted characterizations animate science-based controversy across this wide range of Datagate's texts, I detail how participants, in a mixture of deliberate and unintentional moves, cast one another as villains and victims, as heroes and ordinary janes and joes, and as trustworthy, shady, or somewhere in between. The process was neither neutral nor without implication, for such characterizations influenced assessments of individual integrity, epistemic validity, and the appropriate courses of policy and action. These characterizations drew from and registered, encoded, and sometimes challenged deep cultural assumptions about scientists. Therefore, if we consider the character contests of Datagate as part of a broader process of characterization, then we can observe the interrelations of three distinct concepts—ethos, persona, and voice—and consider how they affect character assessments. More specifically, we can track how prevalent suppositions about the normative behavior of scientists (the scientific *ethos*) cohered into recurrent and relatively stable characterizations of particular types of scientists (scientific *personae*) which, when inflected with the particular lexical and stylistic tendencies of particular speakers (*voice*) colored the meanings, outcomes, and policy responses to this science-based controversy.

This book therefore demonstrates how distinct personae emerge from the cauldron of controversy, and it shows how these personae are collectively crafted and mediated through the speaker-scientists' particular choices and through the representation of the speaker-scientist by others in a process that is amplified and altered through the media as the controversy progresses. In the contentious dramas of publicly ventilated science-based controversies such as Datagate, I argue, credibility does not adhere to particular, historical persons, but rather attaches to constructed personae that emerge in interaction between broader culturally derived stereotypes (ethos) and individual linguistic tendencies (voice). In the mass-mediated public context, it mattered little who the "'data falsifier' Roger Poisson," the "'man in charge' Bernard Fisher," and other players really were, but it mattered a great deal who people said "Roger Poisson," "Bernard Fisher," and "breast cancer patients" were; these constructions in turn affected what counted as trustworthy and actionable knowledge. Our understanding of the controversy will thus have less to do with the bare facts of science per se than with how the facts are animated, challenged, and sustained by rhetorical characterizations, and with how these characterizations, in turn, constrain epistemic, policy, and evaluative judgments and outcomes.[22] None of this is to suggest, however, that the "facts" as humans understand them do not matter, but rather to acknowledge the capacity of rhetoric to foster judgments about the world around us in cases where knowledge is contingent, questioned, or uncertain.

In addition to shaping understanding and constraining action, characterizations divulge key communal norms—in this case, about science and its relationship to broader stakeholders. My study therefore suggests that if scientific personae represent key collective concerns of an epoch, then tracking the personae that animated Datagate can reveal normative assumptions about science and its relationships to and broader antagonisms with publics and stakeholders.[23] Moreover, because scientists are not the only players who participate in science-based controversies, I also consider the characterizations of the advocates and politicians who weighed in during the debates and outline the rhetorical dilemmas they faced in challenging the scientific orthodoxy. By unraveling the contested constellation of characters who animated and sustained Datagate, I illuminate the complex contours of character and reason and thus address an important but under-scrutinized dimension of the rhetorical processes involved when varied publics come together to make sense of complicated scientific matters. Ultimately, I maintain that studying the rhetorically constituted characters that animate science-based controversies is both a primary task for understanding the influence of science in the contemporary life-world and also for tracking the tangled relationship between the norms of democracy and public life and the specialized knowledge found in technical realms like science.

Because one of the core assumptions of a rhetorical perspective is that rhetoric arises from unique constellations of sociohistorical circumstances, its study must attend to the complexion of particular cases. Rhetorician S. Michael Halloran has observed that "particular cases of scientific rhetoric will exhibit their own peculiarities" and that "[a] detailed understanding of the rhetoric of science will have to include some sense of the permissible range or variation."[24] Following Halloran and others, I seek to analyze the rhetoric of a controversy that had profound implications for patients, scientific practitioners, and the general citizenry and limn the range of possible rhetorical choices available to participants in the controversy. But more than that, I analyze the Datagate scandal with the aim of assessing how the rhetorical construction of scientific character influenced the understandings and resolution of a seminal science-based controversy. In the following section, I offer a fuller account of the contours of this case, revealing both its significance to the scientific community and the lives of breast cancer patients as well as its broad entanglements of trust and character.

ANATOMY OF DATAGATE

In 1977, when Roger Poisson directed a staff member to use a blob of correction fluid to modify a patient's breast cancer biopsy date on a research chart, he likely did not envision the worldwide wrath his actions would incur some seventeen years later. When uncovered by breast cancer patients, advocates, politicians, journalists, and fellow medical professionals in the spring of 1994, what had then seemed trivial turned tragic. After all, in the late 1970s the future for cancer research burgeoned with possibility. President Nixon's "War on Cancer" and the women's health movement had spurred a breast cancer research funding bonanza, and Poisson had teamed up with brash American researcher Dr. Bernard Fisher to fight the "dread disease" with lumpectomy and radiation.[25]

Fisher's role in the drama began in the late 1950s, when he headed the NSABP, which he would eventually headquarter at the University of Pittsburgh in 1970.[26] Under Fisher's direction, the NSABP grew from a loose association of doctors interested in tumor and spread into one of the largest and most respected multisite clinical research programs in North America.[27] During the 1970s Fisher joined breast cancer reformers to promote the idea that cancer spread systemically through the lymphatic system rather than outward from the tumor site. This theory supported the view that lumpectomy with follow-up irradiation was the best intervention for early-stage breast cancers and bucked the idea that the Halsted radical mastectomy was the most sensible way to save lives. Scientific justification for lumpectomy with radiation was significant because it upended Halsted's long-standing surgical practice. Advanced in 1882 by celebrated surgeon William Stewart Halsted, the total or radical mastectomy, as it was also called, entailed removal of nipples and breast tissue, their underlying chest muscles, and lymph nodes under the armpit. B-06's finding in support of lumpectomy with radiation as treatment for early-stage cancer thus rendered Halsted's extensive removal of flesh and its ensuing pain, psychological scars, and physical deformation unnecessary. Women with cancer could keep their breasts! To promote this view, Fisher appeared in *Ladies' Home Journal,* visited talk shows, and embarked on a national speaking tour. His coauthored 1985 and 1989 *New England Journal of Medicine* publications detailing the findings of NSABP's B-06 trial were highly regarded.[28] They cemented Fisher's reputation as a reformer of women's health care and affirmed the NSABP's centrality in the annals of U.S. biomedical research. By the early 1990s, Fisher and the NSABP's research continued to flourish; the NSABP conducted an ever-growing array of clinical trials, both preventive and curative, and the group gleaned increasing research dollars, momentum, and prestige.

Back in Montreal, Poisson continued to enroll women into the group's increasingly prominent research. But on at least six occasions, Poisson or his staff altered or left blank the dates of diagnosis on the charts of women enrolled in NSABP's much-celebrated B-06 trial. In 1982, for instance, he, or an office member following his suggestion, changed a patient's diagnosis date from "3/1/82" to "3/11/82."[29] The ten-day difference meant the woman met the date requirement for participating in the research protocol when technically she should not have been allowed to participate. This and similar discrepancies sat undiscovered in research records at Saint-Luc Hospital in Montreal for well over a decade. In the meantime, Poisson recruited swelling numbers of subjects to clinical research, ran a healthy practice, and en-

joyed an increasingly higher placement in the coauthor list on NSABP publications. Few had any reason to assume that his data was awry, routine
audits uncovered no problems, and business continued as usual until June
1990, when an NSABP assistant made an inadvertent but disturbing discovery in the NSABP's Pittsburgh office: Poisson had changed the charts.

Before journalist John Crewdson's stunning announcement of Poisson's
"fraud" in the *Chicago Tribune* in mid-March 1994, only NSABP staff, governmental oversight officials, and a few key insiders knew that Fisher's co-
investigator Roger Poisson had confessed to research misconduct in the
nation's premier breast cancer research.[30] More specifically, the physician-
investigator had admitted to falsifying 115 separate pieces of data in 99 patient records used in 14 NSABP trials between 1977 and 1991.[31] Six of
these falsifications occurred in B-06, and because B-06 was the largest study
of lumpectomy's efficacy, changes to its findings potentially affected international treatment recommendations, raising the stakes for many patients
and health-care providers.[32] Poisson's six B-06 transgressions involved altering diagnosis and surgery dates on study forms to make otherwise ineligible patients eligible to participate in the NIH-funded research.[33] An investigation headed by the U.S. Office of Research Integrity (ORI) found
Poisson guilty of misconduct.[34] ORI reported their finding, along with fourteen others, on page 33,831 of the *Federal Register*, a publication for government employees.[35] Poisson's case appeared ninth in a list of incidents of scientific misconduct, occurring between notice of a doctor who plagiarized
parts of a grant application and news of a master's student who fabricated
and falsified data in her laboratory notebook. According to journalist Kathy
Sawyer, the Department of Health and Human Services (HHS) had issued
a press release about the *Federal Register* notice the week before its release,
but ORI's public relations office "stripped and toned down" the language describing the findings, and they did not link Poisson's case to the landmark
lumpectomy study.[36] ORI's finding thus passed with mere murmurs until
Crewdson's dramatic headline nearly four years after the initial discovery of
discrepant data.

Acting on a tip from a Washington insider, Crewdson broke the story;
a frenzy of activity followed his intervention into the high-stakes life-and-
death world of breast cancer research. Just months before, Fisher had enjoyed "an unchallenged spot in the medical pantheon."[37] He had received
virtually every major medical award for his research. Now, after receiving
publicity that a researcher under his direction had falsified data used in federally funded breast cancer treatment studies, his career was in tatters. He
was unceremoniously forced to resign from his position at the University of

Pittsburgh, where he had worked for more than three decades, and was required to step down as chair of the NSABP. Eventually, bibliographic entries for 148 of his scientific articles were, inappropriately it would turn out, marked with the tag "scientific misconduct—data to be reanalyzed" in the widely disseminated electronic indexes *Medline, Cancerlit,* and *Physicians' Data Query.*[38] Even more threatening than allegations of scientific misconduct, however, were charges made by breast cancer advocacy groups that Fisher had quashed reports of tamoxifen-induced endometrial cancer deaths in the highly celebrated $68 million breast cancer prevention trial (BCPT) also under his direction.[39] This first-ever breast cancer prevention trial, "one of the most ambitious and controversial" studies that the National Cancer Institute (NCI) had ever funded, involved eleven thousand healthy women at risk of developing breast cancer, half of whom were taking the cancer drug tamoxifen.[40] Fisher was eventually cleared of any wrongdoing related to either the B-06 trial or the BCPT study, but in the argle-bargle of the Datagate imbroglio, the early fallout was severe. In response to public outcry and political pressure concerning these various charges, the NCI suspended all NSABP clinical trials in March 1994.

Sensing, if not also fueling, the trouble to come, other newspapers picked up the themes of Crewdson's report, prompting front-page stories in the *New York Times,* the *Washington Post,* and the *Los Angeles Times.* Heightened media attention pressured oversight officials to maintain the image that they were doing everything possible to root out fraud and solve the problem. Accordingly, they ratcheted up scrutiny of NSABP records. Within a week, Fisher received an urgent call from Richard Ungerleider, NCI's chief of clinical investigations, stating that NSABP paperwork revealed problems at Louisiana State University and Tulane. Ungerleider ordered Fisher to dispatch his top people to conduct audits by the following Monday and to suspend all trials there.[41] When top aides Lawrence Wickerham and Walter Cronin went to Louisiana to conduct the audits, Fisher persevered without key assistants to face the onslaught of questions and requests. According to *Pittsburgh Post-Gazette* reporters Mackenzie Carpenter and Steve Twedt, University of Pittsburgh officials "had just learned about the Montreal fraud through the *Chicago Tribune* article because Fisher, who had known about it for three years, had not told them."[42] They called a meeting with Fisher. It was around the time of this meeting that Fisher, in consultation with his university-hired advisers, made the fateful decision to "do nothing publicly and to wait and see what happened next."[43]

What happened next, on March 20, was that requests for information started inundating Fisher's office. "The fax machine started spewing and never let up," Fisher told the *Pittsburgh Post-Gazette*. "We were working 18 hours a day . . . We were trying to fulfill these orders, and it was just chaos."[44] Just when the situation seemed impossible, it got even worse. Officials discovered problems with data from St. Mary's Hospital in Montreal, problems they believed NSABP officials had previously identified. On March 28, NCI's Michael Friedman, then director of cancer therapy evaluation, telephoned Fisher in Pittsburgh. A recounting of that colorful conversation, based on Fisher's recollection, appeared in the *Post-Gazette*:

> "We've found out you knew about the St. Mary's audit, and didn't do anything," Freidman told Fisher angrily.
>
> Fisher said his staff had never told him about the St. Mary's audit until it was discovered by the NCI official. That didn't placate Friedman.
>
> "This will tear down research all across the country," Friedman said, over Fisher's protests that he didn't know what Friedman was talking about . . .
>
> "You're finished, Bernie!" Friedman yelled. "You got (screwed) by your staff. You're out!"[45]

A March 29 letter from the NCI to the University of Pittsburgh ordered the university to remove Fisher as head of the NSABP due to a "litany of NSABP failures."[46] A University of Pittsburgh press release dated the same day quoted Fisher as "requesting administrative leave from the chair of NSABP so that I can continue my investigations . . . which are so important to the women of this country."[47] For a man whose professional life had revolved almost exclusively around the University of Pittsburgh and the NSABP, this must have been a stunning blow. Meanwhile, the NCI placed the NSABP on probation and ordered the group to suspend new patient accruals and to conduct extensive audits. At stake was the forfeiture of NCI grants to NSABP totaling $22 million a year, $10 million of which went directly to the university.[48]

This dizzying crescendo of events prompted congressman John Dingell's (D-MI) call for House Subcommittee on Oversight and Investigations hearings for April and June 1994. One unnamed spokesman for the House subcommittee said that the purpose of the hearing was to determine "how the system collapsed from beginning to end."[49] Fisher's initial encounter with Representative Dingell proved, in the words of one journalist, "withering."[50] With millions of dollars of taxpayer-funded research grants—not to mention breast cancer patients' sense of security—suddenly on the line, the agencies that stood to lose them were looking for a ritual scapegoat, and some observers believed they had found their man in then-seventy-five-year-old Fisher. The June 24, 1994, issue of the *Cancer Letter*, one of the nation's most widely circulated professional oncology newsletters, described the hearing as "tragic for Bernard Fisher" and announced: "Fisher Unable to Answer Key Questions."[51]

The hearing was also heartrending for breast cancer patients who had placed their faith in—and staked their lives on—NSABP research. A month before Fisher's testimony, Washington-based advocate and breast cancer survivor Jill Lea Sigal also testified before Dingell's subcommittee about how news of data falsification in NSABP research had affected her. Tearfully, the thirty-two-year-old woman, whom Dingell described as "victimized" by breast cancer, recounted her "anger and outrage that a doctor could possibly engage in such gross scientific fraud."[52] In the view of Daniel S. Greenberg in the British medical journal the *Lancet*, Sigal "emotionally sounded the theme of betrayal."[53] "How many women must now wonder, as I do every day, if they will die because they have made the wrong decision?" she asked the subcommittee, noting that she had based her breast cancer treatment decision on the now reputationally challenged NSABP research.[54] In so doing, Sigal had joined tens of thousands of American women who opted to have a breast-conserving lumpectomy with follow-up radiation instead of the potentially disfiguring breast-removing mastectomy that NSABP research had demonstrated was unnecessary for early-stage breast cancers. "Mr. Chairman," she asserted, "there seems to be no end to the fraud and deception. As a result of the National Cancer Institute's behavior in this manner, I now question other policies of the National Cancer Institute, including its policy that women under the age of 50 should not get a mammogram unless they are at high risk."[55] Television newscasts amplified her testimony; newscasters intoned details about the "chilling case of greed and ego."[56] Trust hung in the balance; lives were on the line. Harmon Eyre of the ACS observed that "this is creating a substantial problem of trust and uncertainty . . . Women are challenging whether or not they had the right treatment, and doctors are concerned about how to respond."[57]

To "get to the bottom of the matter," Dingell, then chair of the Oversight Subcommittee of the House Committee on Energy and Commerce, called key institutional representatives to testify in Washington, DC. A second-generation career politician, Dingell was a formidable opponent for Fisher and the other scientists he called to Capitol Hill. Dubbed the "Dark Knight of Science" by one commentator, Dingell believed that the scientific community had "been treated as a sacred cow for far too long" and needed to become more accountable to the public.[58] He was well known for displaying the investigative zeal of a former prosecutor; his efforts to bring big science to task through well-publicized hearings had become so notorious that by the early 1990s they were dubbed the "Dingellization" of science; they were both widely feared and roundly criticized by members of the scientific community.[59] Dingell's subcommittee had jurisdiction over the National Institutes of Health; its National Cancer Institute had funded Fisher's NSABP research. Fisher was never himself accused of any data falsification; he was merely charged with poor oversight, but his insistent denials of wrongdoing were met with a fusillade of alleged failures from officials at the University of Pittsburgh and various federal agencies. Dingell thus opened the June hearing with a list of five failures on the part of Fisher, the University of Pittsburgh, and the NCI. He characterized the failures as "multiple and serious," yet "only a part of a long story" involving "serious and chronic problems of missing and misrepresented data."[60] The unfolding tale of misdeeds and miscommunication in federally funded breast cancer research undermined confidence in clinical trials, raised ethical questions for the medical community, frustrated researchers who felt like they had acted on good faith, terrified women who had used NSABP studies as the basis for making treatment decisions, and heightened the anxiety of patients facing breast cancer in the wake of the controversy.[61]

In the cool light of history, and from a technical/scientific viewpoint, the B-06 controversy pivoted on just six pieces of discrepant data of a total number of 354 cases that Roger Poisson was responsible for overseeing at Saint-Luc Hospital.[62] Because these 354 cases formed part of 2,163 patients enrolled in the study, the complete removal of all 354 of Poisson's patients would not have changed the findings of the study, as the *Lancet* underscored: "the trial's conclusions were unaltered on reanalysis when either these 6 patients or all 354 entered by Poisson were eliminated from the calculations."[63] From the perspective of many onlookers and breast cancer advocates, however, Poisson's six alterations in B-06 and other deceptions comprised more than a whiff of wider irregularities that called the entire federal research enterprise into question.[64] For many observers, the issue with Datagate was that it "smacked of a scientific cover-up."[65] "I take no comfort, no comfort whatsoever," said Jill Sigal, "from the fact that the Institute that swept the fraud under the rug for three years now claims to have conducted a re-analysis of the study and maintains that the findings are still valid."[66] Sigal's comments disclose how the Datagate controversy is only a symptom of the larger political struggles of its time, for it exposes tensions between cancer advocates and physicians, big science and politics, and activists and consumers.

Despite its nuances, the issues raised by Datagate extend beyond the confines of this particular case. Indeed, a recurrent stream of science-based controversies potentially disrupts the delicate balance of belief that undergirds science. Contests over the claims of climate research; the findings of genetic studies; the discovery of possible misconduct; and the potential perils of drinking, obesity, and smoking, to name but a few, routinely make news, comprising a recurrent genre of mass-mediated science coverage, most of which is driven by character, contest, and controversy. For instance, headlines such as "Criticism of a Gender Theory, and a Scientist under Siege," "Most Science Studies Appear to Be Tainted by Sloppy Analysis," or "Health Officials Cleared of Vaccine Misconduct" index the interaction of character and knowledge in public sphere communication about science.[67] Regardless of whether the dissensus that typifies these recurrent controversies is fictitious, exaggerated, or more or less faithfully presented, its mediated reportage forms a primary point of contact between many citizens and scientific claims.

As both Datagate and these recent headlines suggest, science occupies an increasingly visible and consequential part of our public sphere. Yet as Judy Segal and Alan Richardson have noted, "When science speaks, it speaks through scientists."[68] In order to understand the rhetorical situations that call scientists to speak on controversial matters in the public sphere and the situations in which their character as professional scientists and private citizens becomes a matter of broader debate, we need to begin by analyzing the particular instances in which this happened on both descriptive and evaluative levels, and that is the central aim of this book. It is important to note, however, that by choosing to focus on character in Datagate, this book does not offer a comprehensive history of the case, nor does it attempt to offer a definitive account of the labyrinthine turn of events or a philosophical treatise on the components of trust. Those tasks I leave to historians, cultural chroniclers, and philosophers. Instead, my purview in the forthcoming chapters concerns public arguments that praise and defend particular scientists and interested stakeholders, those places where the characters of principal players are cultivated, contested, and reshaped in public and technical discourse.[69] I therefore offer but one interpretation of a complicated, highly contested case in the hope that it will spark further consideration of how trust, rhetoric, character, science, and its varied stakeholders commingle.

Chapter 1 offers the theoretical and historical background for the remainder of the study. I open by presenting a three-part scheme for analyzing character construction in science-based controversies. More specifically, I detail how ethos, persona, and voice—three interrelated but conceptually distinct terms with origins that span rhetoric, drama, literary studies, and sociology—together reveal the complex workings of character in science-based controversies. I then situate Datagate within a broader context of twentieth-century biomedical research, including the rise of randomized clinical trials, increasing concerns about research integrity, the growing patient autonomy movement, and the changing face of breast cancer surgery. These contexts reveal the rhetorical constraints faced by the scientists, politicians, patients, and activists whose voices contributed to Datagate.

Chapter 2 investigates the Janus-faced representations of Dr. Roger Poisson, the Montreal-based physician-researcher whose data alterations triggered what Canadians called "*L'Affaire Poisson.*" Drawing on newspaper, magazine, and medical journal accounts in the United States and Canada, this chapter tracks the battle over the bifurcated representations of Poisson as a beneficent healer and as a career-minded fraud. Janus, god of passages, portals, and doorways, is an appropriate figure to signify the two characterizations of a man caught between dueling worlds—the mythos of the ancient and humane art of healing, the equally potent myth of the purity of scientific research, complicated as it is by the constraints of bureaucratized research. These two personae, these masks onto which Poisson's actions are projected, highlighted a tension that continues to haunt contemporary biomedicine, one that is further complicated by the politics driving big science—namely, the conflict between the physician who treats and the researcher who studies. In scrutinizing the contested characterizations of Roger Poisson, we learn what is gained and lost in the present clinical trials system with its blurred division between those who treat and those who study. Thus, my analysis of ethos, persona, and voice in chapter 2 explains the rhetorical and ethical liabilities of a role conflict inherent in the physician-researcher.

Chapter 3 tracks the competing personae of Dr. Bernard Fisher, the "man in charge" of the then-tarnished breast cancer study, and chronicles how his four competing personae vied for legitimacy and acceptance in professional, political, and public spheres in the early months of the controversy. Drawing on documents from the 1950s to the present, I begin by charting Fisher's rising prominence in twentieth-century breast cancer research. Here, I reveal his challenge to the surgical orthodoxy and trace his relentless efforts to persuade colleagues of the necessity of clinical trials. As time went on, Fisher, and then others, scripted his accomplishments in terms of one of the most enduring scientific personae—the scientific revolutionary. Moving forward to the Datagate controversy that shook the foundation of Fisher's work, I then analyze challenges to the revolutionary persona that emerged during the scandal. More specifically, I sort through the inner relations and implications of the personae of the scientific revolutionary, the reluctant apologist, the beleaguered bureaucrat, and eventually, the vindicated visionary. Each of these personae carried different potential for both Fisher's reputation and the ethos of science; each revealed a different face of the challenges inherent in big science.

Having laid out the foundation for the study in chapter 1 and having addressed the two key scientist-physicians involved in the imbroglio in chapters 2 and 3, chapter 4 then addresses the division between science and its stakeholders by examining breast cancer patients' and advocates' participation in Datagate. This chapter explores the recurrent characterizations of patients, activists, advocates, and politicians who struggled to make sense of what Datagate meant in terms of women's health care in general and breast cancer treatment in particular. Although these characters arguably had the most at stake in the controversy, they often found themselves spoken for by the other players. Chapter 4 begins by chronicling women's participation in breast cancer research over the course of the twentieth century and concludes by considering rhetorical strategies for intervening in biomedical research. Along the way, it analyzes the implications of several dominant characterizations of breast cancer advocates and the politicians who weighed in as their "protectors": the knowledge consumer, the victim/subject of science, and the knowledge partner. Although these characters are dynamic and overlapping, I conclude that the latter affords the greatest possibilities for effecting change in biomedical research.

Chapter 5 transports the lessons of Datagate into the broader realm of the recurrent skirmishes over scientific integrity that invariably spawn headlines and fuel protracted disputes. It explores how the stock personae of Fisher and Poisson represent some of the key tensions faced by scientists who may be called to account for their actions in the public sphere, while the personae of politicians and advocates similarly suggest the difficulties inherent in attempts to police science from the outside. I conclude by reflecting on what Datagate reveals about rhetorical agency, both for scientists and for citizens. Here, I discuss rhetorical strategies for citizen and scientist engagement with scientific practices that can meaningfully account for the interests of those affected by the research. In short, I offer a road map for a recharacterization of participation in science-based controversy. *Scientific Characters* concludes by arguing that sustained reconsideration of the interrelatedness of character and knowledge, of trust and truth, can augment studies of science-based controversies wherein scientists and members of various publics deliberate about matters that affect them all.

More than thirty-five years have passed since Yaron Ezrahi, writing in the inaugural volume of *Science Studies* in 1971, apologized lest readers find "The Political Resources of American Science," his title and topic, "somewhat perverse, if not entirely heretical," since the "traditional ethos of science emphasized 'a complete separation between science and politics.'"[70] Today, few commentators would argue that science and politics were anything but intimately connected. Accordingly, this book seeks to enrich our understanding of how science-based controversies play out in political realms by demonstrating how rhetorically forged constructions of character can animate, complicate, and contribute to the resolution of these debates. In a time when public life is awash in scientific knowledge, when various stakeholders see science both as salvation and as spreader of wreckage and waste, when scientific disputes routinely appear amid an endless barrage of news, understanding the inextricable links between rhetoric and character, science and publics, and trust and truth is a paramount task indeed.

1

Scientists under Scrutiny: The Centrality of Character in Science-Based Controversy

When the Datagate controversy was but two weeks old, breast cancer patients and the broader medical establishment were still reeling from the news of Roger Poisson's tarnished data when auditors uncovered evidence of additional flaws at a second NSABP research site. As if the discovery of falsified data at one site were not damaging enough, the whiff of wider irregularities triggered a crisis of confidence. "Erosion of Public Trust?" asked the *Cancer Letter* as it reported a discrepant date found on a patient chart at St. Mary's Hospital in Montreal.[1] Cindy Pearson, then director of the National Women's Health Network (NWHN), told the *Cancer Letter* that "to find out that the NSABP can't even guarantee the quality of record-keeping and adherence to this trial, this adds insult to injury."[2] Meanwhile, Fran Visco, president of the National Breast Cancer Coalition (NBCC), explained, "I think the public trust has been eroded to such an extent that what is needed now is an independent investigation."[3] While National Cancer Institute and NSABP officers tried to assure broader publics that there was "no cause for concern," the *Cancer Letter,* Pearson, and Visco attested to a fraying of trust in the institutions charged with overseeing research that affected patients' lives. Their words indexed the broader issue raised in this book's introduction: science relies on the testimony of strangers; doubts about the trustworthiness of such testimony undermine confidence in the underlying system and expose the underlying norms of science to broader scrutiny by members of various publics in ways that invoke, challenge, or revise widespread stereotypes about science.[4]

The terms *science* and *scientist* conjure commanding images of purity, precision, and, above all, disinterestedness in the outcomes of research. As philosopher Richard Rorty once observed, "'science,' 'rationality,' 'objectivity' and 'truth' are bound up with one another."[5] "Science," he explained "is thought of as offering 'hard,' 'objective' truth."[6] Rorty's comments reflect widespread stereotypes suggesting that the character of individual scientists should not affect the outcomes of scientific practice. The particular people who populate science, in this view, do not matter so much as their abandonment of human foibles in service of the loftier pursuit of dispassionate, disinterested, and objective knowledge. Science studies scholar Brian Martin captured the thrust of this view when he explained, "Scientific truths are not supposed to be tainted by interests, which is why scientific knowledge is portrayed as rising above the limitations of the system that created it."[7] Although competing images of science certainly abound, Progressive-era ideas about science nevertheless consolidated an image of scientists as "models of seriousness, caution, and neutrality, whose detachment guaranteed the reliability of their investigators"—a vision that bears resonance today.[8] Indeed, "to argue for the importance, even the centrality, of the personal dimension in late modern technoscience," writes science studies scholar Steven Shapin, "is directly to confront a sensibility that defines almost all academic, and probably much lay, thought about late modern culture."[9]

Given this tendency to view scientists as neutral, objective, and unbiased, it is therefore not surprising that when widespread agreement over knowledge claims exists, the *character* of science passes without comment. But when the epistemic status of knowledge claims is uncertain, threatened, or tarnished, speculation about the character of science and the character of particular scientists looms large. As experts and nonexperts weigh in on the validity of the disputed knowledge claims, they try to persuade one another about the trustworthiness of scientific arguments, methods, and persons. The rhetoric produced in these exchanges is akin to what sociologist of science Thomas F. Gieryn calls a *credibility contest*: a "chronic feature of the social scene," in which "bearers of discrepant truths push their wares wrapped in assertions of objectivity, efficacy, precision, reliability, authenticity, predictability, sincerity, desirability, and tradition."[10] In rhetorical terms, credibility contests involve attempts to convince others of the integrity of individual actions, of the moral uprightness of particular scientists, and whether or not the character of the arguer makes a difference to the status of his or her knowledge claims, thus revealing the snug relationship between trust and truth, character and knowledge, and the language choices that facilitate their construction.

During Datagate, scientists, administrators, institutional representatives, activists and advocates, patients, caretakers, and health-care workers wrangled over the integrity of NSABP research and, by extension, over the validity

of federally funded science. Many of these people also fought to retain, re-
gain, and rehabilitate others' estimations of their character and credibility
while simultaneously trying to maintain the epistemic authority of science,
the "legitimate power to define, describe, and explain bounded domains of
reality."[11] As scientists, administrators, politicians, and patients struggled to
make sense of events, they enacted particular rhetorical strategies designed
to protect their interests and to enable them to process competing arguments about or related to science. However, in attempting to bolster their
own reputations, the key players often damaged the credibility of themselves and others, for their less-than-elegant public rhetoric, shared in a dynamic and unstable process that reshaped the contours of scientific practice, often left them seeming less, not more, credible.[12] Yet trust, as Harriet
Zuckerman noted, "is central for the system of science," and trust, we shall
discover later in this chapter, depends deeply on perceptions of character.[13]

By outlining a rhetorical perspective on character and by situating Datagate within its historical milieu, this chapter details the theoretical and con-
textual foundation for my study. In what follows, I advance a three-part
framework for analyzing contested characterizations, one that is perhaps
versatile enough to illuminate character struggles in many social dramas
but that I apply specifically to the vagaries of a science-based controversy
wherein widespread stereotypes about science influenced expectations about
scientific character. My framework for analyzing character draws from and
extends two key concepts from the classical tradition, one long associated
with rhetoric and the other a venerated part of the literary tradition in Western education. These concepts are ethos and persona; to them I add a third
concept called voice. Admittedly, ethos, persona, and voice encompass contested definitions and wide usage discrepancies, but the triad shares a concern for rhetorically constituted identity and hints at the difference between
the actual self and the self constructed through public discourse.

I begin the chapter by situating my three-part method for analyzing
character within the rhetoric of science, and then I explain how it can produce nuanced, qualitative interpretations of how character contests play out
in the cauldron of controversy. Because science-based controversies stem
from particular sociohistorical contingencies, I then review the forces that
gave rise to Datagate, thus setting the stage for the chapters to come. Ultimately, I hope to offer a rhetorical perspective on an old observation that has
since been muted by the rise of big science with its imprimatur of impersonal-
ity: In 1938 Dr. David Lindsay Watson made the seemingly simple point,
as the title of his book proclaimed, that "Scientists Are Human."[14] Watson
maintained that aspects of the scientist's "mental life" influence "the trust-

worthiness of his product, and in particular make the findings of science subject to weakness and passion like other human constructions."[15] Somewhere along the way, Watson's message became supplanted by a vision of an impersonal, institutionalized and corporatized, neutral and objective science. In the pages that follow, we shall revisit the human dimension of science and the role of rhetoric in forging character.

THE RHETORIC OF SCIENCE

Because character is mediated through language, a chasm separates a living person from representations of that person's character. What we mainly encounter in public life are selves projected and (re)negotiated discursively, a fact that suggests the importance of the rhetorical tradition for understanding character construction in science-based controversy. In seeking to untangle Datagate's disparate constructions of character, this study springs from both a long tradition of rhetorical criticism and a multidisciplinary initiative known as the rhetoric of science, which seeks to explain the role of persuasion in science and science-related communication. Generally speaking, rhetoric has concerned itself with the practice and analysis of strategic language; a major task of rhetorical scholarship has been to explicate the "available means of persuasion" in particular cases.[16] Historically, these cases were drawn from the province of public and political affairs, but rhetoricians of science, starting in the 1970s, turned their analytic energies to the persuasive dimensions of scientific texts, contexts, processes, and practices to demonstrate how rhetoric is involved in some of the most elemental processes of science.[17] Randy Allen Harris has defined the rhetoric of science as "the study of how scientists persuade and dissuade each other and the rest of us about nature, the study of how scientists argue in the making of knowledge."[18] Yet because scientific life affects and is affected by more than just scientists, I expand his definition to consider persuasion both in the conduct of science and in its circulation in public life—that is, to examine both the rhetoric *of* scientists and the rhetoric *about* scientists and science, which may or may not emanate from voices steeped in scientific subject positions. I therefore follow Charles Alan Taylor in examining "the functional use of discourse to define, redefine, even to deconstruct, the implicit boundaries of those social practices we consider scientific."[19] In the broadest sense, I am concerned with how rhetoric is implicated in the collective cultural processes by which we come to understand science.[20]

The rhetoric of science forms part of a broader multidisciplinary movement organized under the umbrella of "science studies," which situate scientific practices in historical, cultural, philosophical, social, and political contexts.[21] Although they are methodologically diverse and philosophically heterogeneous, science studies represent an effort to replace the mythos of scientific objectivism and boundless progress with sustained consideration of how social processes shape and are shaped by science. Whereas other branches of science studies consider the historical, philosophical, and sociocultural dimensions of science, the rhetoric of science focuses on how language affects scientific processes and understandings. Scholarship in the rhetoric of science assumes that "science and, by implication, scientific knowledge are social constructions which are given presence in rhetorical discourse."[22] Such a perspective does not imply that science swims in a squishy sea of relativity; rather, it asserts that science, like all forms of knowledge, is "a complex, multidimensional phenomenon based on the aggregation of many nondefinitive pieces of evidence and experience."[23]

Accordingly, scholarship in the rhetoric of science generally maintains that rhetoric is deeply implicated in the process of coming-to-know. A slogan that captures this sentiment is Robert L. Scott's maxim that "rhetoric is epistemic."[24] Applied to science, the idea that rhetoric is bound up in coming-to-know means the only way we can understand natural phenomena is through language, which indelibly shapes our understanding of phenomena and primes our responses to them. As Lawrence Prelli notes, "Rhetorical acts present allegations about what is; they symbolically address contentions about how we should name, pattern, or define experiences and thereby make those experiences meaningful."[25] A rhetorical perspective therefore licenses studies of how rhetoric is involved in knowledge production, how it fosters identity formation, and how it coordinates the realm of human affairs. It assumes that science, as a complex, linguistically mediated, heterogeneous set of institutional practices, is a contentious and argument-driven affair, brimming with the possibilities and perils of human involvement. Yet it also acknowledges that science, shrouded in a deep cloak of presumed objectivism, is both enabled and constrained by widespread stereotypes about its ideals and capacities. Thus, when rhetoricians study discourses of and about science, their dominant approach comprises a method known as rhetorical criticism, a humanistic and interpretive act whereby the critic "takes up a text and re-circulates it, that is [the critic] 'says' or 'does' that text differently, and asks the listener or reader to re-understand and re-evaluate the text, to see and judge it in new ways suggested by the critic."[26] My study of Datagate takes up the texts of this controversy and refracts them through the lens of rhetorically constituted character, for the plethora of press releases, public appearances, and journal correspondence generated by key players in NSABP Datagate teem with competing characterizations that were amplified through reports in the mass media. These characterizations and the story lines into which they are embedded have consequences; they can perpetuate or alleviate personal stigmatization and rehabilitate or tarnish reputation, open up or obscure lines of policy and action, and reveal the interconnectedness of those who together confronted the harsh realities of breast cancer.

A RHETORICAL PERSPECTIVE ON CHARACTER

Richard Harvey Brown has noted that "the narrative character of science lies not in a story completed but in a story being told, a story constantly being struggled over and adjusted."[27] When news media, medical journals, health-care professionals, and advocates and citizens spoke in public about Datagate, they enacted strategic selection and framing of key developments, which implanted characterizations of its players into stories. Shapin has observed that in science, "stories about people and their personal characteristics, their virtues and vices, travel around the community with remarkable speed and efficiency."[28] In the news media, this process comprised what James S. Ettema and Theodore L. Glasser have called "news-as-narrative," which underscores the broader orientational power of narrative.[29] The narrative form of the news story is, for Ettema and Glasser, "an 'instrument' of comprehension and cognition."[30] Yet more than presenting facts and events in a recognizable and understandable package, narrative, following Hayden White, is also "an instrument for the assertion of moral authority," meaning that stories organize reality into ways that invite participation in moral order.[31] Those who encounter narratives can make judgments about the version of morality implied in a story. Moreover, these audiences can make assessments about the morality of a story's protagonists and antagonists; particular constructions of the key players in the controversy thus encourage certain assessments of integrity—and in the case of science-based controversy, believability—over others. As participants in controversy weigh in, they narrativize events in ways that characterize key players, which encode normative understandings about who the scientist is and should be. Three dimensions of character in particular—*ethos, persona,* and *voice*—illuminate this process, and compel detailed analyses of the complicated workings of character construction.

Ethos

When the credibility of scientists is on the line, participants look to communal understandings of science—the scientific ethos—as a means of assessing if their faith is misplaced. While science studies scholars have a relatively recent but elaborated literature on the scientific ethos, scholars in rhetoric and composition studies have been mulling over the nuances of ethos for centuries. Marshall Alcorn observed that "although our understanding of *ethos* has changed over the years, one feature remains constant: thinkers as diverse as Aristotle and Kenneth Burke agree that often it is not a person's *ideas* but a person's *character* that changes people."[32] Aristotle placed character at the center of persuasion when he discussed "finding out how to make our hearers take the required view of our own characters."[33] Although I use Aristotle as a point of departure for reinvigorating an older sense of ethos, and thus do not regard my book as Aristotelian, his influence on contemporary notions of the concept merits review. Conceived in Aristotle's imagining as "persuasion through the character of the speaker," ethos can often propel scientific knowledge.[34] A scientist who is well known and widely respected can advance her knowledge claims with more ease than one who is unknown or mistrusted—regardless of the actual content of the claims each makes. For example, celebrity scientists such as Stephen Hawking or James Watson command more media access than unknown laboratory workers; thus, they enjoy a larger audience for and circulation of their ideas.

Two senses of the ancient concept of ethos illuminate the connection between speakers and their communities. The first addresses the character of the individual speaker. The second represents "the spirit or group character of a broader community of speakers."[35] These two senses interpenetrate because communal values supply the means to assess an individual's ethos. For example, the shared values comprising the Progressive-era vision of scientists as serious, cautious, and neutral contain a normative vision that provides the criteria by which to judge scientists. In the Aristotelian scheme that has dominated scholarly discussion, ethos is one of three artistic proofs that, along with pathos and logos, a speaker can use as a mode of persuasion.[36] Whereas logos involves the strategic use of reason in language, and pathos stirs the emotions, ethos is an appeal to the character of the speaker. As Aristotle's *Rhetoric* suggests, "persuasion is achieved by the speaker's personal character when the speech is so spoken as to make us think him credible."[37] Moreover, "this kind of persuasion, like the others, should be achieved by what the speaker says, not by what people think of this character before he begins to speak."[38] Two key facets of Aristotelian ethos are embedded in this conception. The first is that ethos is more than the mere reputation that exists before and after a speech; it is derived from actual inventional choices themselves, those created by a speaker in the act of speaking.[39] Ethos, here, is treated as an aspect of the art of finding things to say, something that "in any given case" can be discovered as "an available means of persuasion."[40] The second is that, at least for Aristotle, ethos depends on the *appearance* of credibility or character, on what the audience thinks of a speaker's character, not what his or her character might be from the standpoint of an omniscient observer. Thus, we can distinguish between an Aristotelian sense of ethos, which relies on an appearance of being good, and a Platonic or essentialist sense, which would maintain the necessity of actually being good.[41] It is important to note that the sense of character implied by ethos is grounded in trustworthiness, not in a sense of character based on personality, role, or position (although each of these can affect perceptions of ethos). Audiences are persuaded by speakers they trust so that construction of a good self through language is central to the successful deployment of ethos. In this sense, ethos derives from a rhetor's inventional choices but resides in audience assessments of a speaker's character.

Ethos, however, is more complicated than its Aristotelian rendering. Michael Hyde's recent collection of essays, *The Ethos of Rhetoric,* highlighted the "architectural" function of ethos, the use of language to "build a habitat, a dwelling place, where in moments of moral responsibility people can deliberate and 'know-together' (*con-scientia*) what is, arguably, the 'truth' of some contested matter and what actions should follow in light of the decision needed here."[42] Hyde's collection took its inspiration from the original sense of the term *ethos* as a dwelling point. Charles Chamberlain explained that *ethos* "originally designates 'the places where animals are usually found.'"[43] Chamberlain traced the etymology of the term from Homer and Hesiod through Aristotle, stressing its origins in the domain of animals. One's *ēthea* "form[s] an arena or range in which the animal naturally belongs," a designation that signals habituation, an important concept in terms of Aristotle's later development of the word.[44] We judge character by others' habits. Chamberlain also noted the political use of the term as manifest in Thucydides, wherein *ethos* refers to the idiosyncrasies the people of a particular polis acquire, resulting from their having been raised according to the customs and laws of that polis.[45] Ethos in this view derives from law or custom. By Aristotle's time, "what we are left with," according to Chamberlain, "is a quality of animate beings which is like habit in that it prescribes predictable behavior, but something more in that it cannot easily be 're-habituated.'"[46] We judge habits as somewhat stable, as somehow intrinsic to a person, and yet they are shaped by a communal dwelling place, thus revealing the essential link between ethos and community. Retaining this sense of group identity, I will treat ethos as the widely shared cultural values or implied norms that characterize a group of people.

The prevalent, if not mythical, commonsense understanding of science comprises what have come to be known as the "Mertonian norms" of scientific practice, which are sometimes called the "scientific ethos." Merton defined the ethos of science as "that affectively toned complex of values and norms which is held to be binding on the man of science. These norms are expressed in the form of prescriptions, proscriptions, preferences, and permissions. They are legitimized in terms of institutional values. These imperatives, transmitted by precept and example and reenforced [*sic*] by sanctions are in varying degrees internalized by the scientist, thus fashioning his scientific conscience."[47] Merton's 1942 essay "Normative Structure of Science" identified the norms of science as communism (by which Merton meant something akin to communalism), disinterestedness, organized skepticism, and universality.[48] In this view, scientists build on a collective heritage of science and share their findings with the international community, work without manipulating their research to achieve desired ends, are free to question any view or finding, and conduct science according to impersonal criteria. Commentators have argued that rather than being seen as a description of how scientists actually behave, the Mertonian norms actually represent normative ideals for how science ought to be.[49] Moreover, as science and technology scholar Sheila Jasanoff notes, "Much of the authority of science in the twentieth century rests as well on its success in persuading decision-makers and the public that the Mertonian norms present an accurate picture of the way science 'really works.'"[50] When scientists are called to testify before federal officials, for example, the Mertonian norms of science are often used as a benchmark for assessing the character of individual scientists. They serve as argumentative resources for administrators expressing concern about scientific behavior and for scientists seeking to restore their reputations. Thus, the Mertonian norms represent ideals to which scientists are said to aspire, but the reality, as seen in the case of Datagate, is often messier. In the case of the scientific ethos, Merton's norms provide a convenient starting place for discussion. However, in order to flesh out the implications of this communal sense of ethos, we must first consider how particular social performances of roles impinge on perceptions of character. A second concept, persona, helps to illuminate this dimension of character.

Persona

A notion that is related to but conceptually distinct from character is persona, which derives from a literary or dramatic tradition. In contemporary rhetorical scholarship, persona is underutilized and occasionally conflated with ethos.[51] Rhetorician Robert Alan Brookey noted that "in rhetorical studies, the term *persona* is used rarely enough that it is not even indexed in some of the major overviews of rhetorical history."[52] While *persona* does in fact appear less frequently in rhetorical scholarship than *ethos,* it does arise with periodic frequency, even if rhetorical scholars "have seldom kept *ethos* well located, mixing terms, sometimes using *ethos, persona,* and *voice* as if identical."[53] *Persona* derives from the Latin for "mask" or "theatrical mask," such as that worn on stage by Roman actors and by their Greek predecessors, whose term was *prosōpon.*[54] The tragic mask, the ancestral mask, or the death mask embody this notion. Yet the etymology of the term *persona* reveals "one of the most complex histories known to philologists."[55] The late sociologist Marcel Mauss speculated that the reconstruction of *persona* "from *per/sonare,* the mask through (*per*) which the voice (of the actor) sounds," may be retrospective fancy.[56] Nonetheless, Roman rhetorical education advanced *fictio personae* as a master trope. Students were directed to animate a theme with the addition of a character and his or her motivation. Together, these were woven into narratives with students playing the role of their particular character.[57] This process produced "a kind of ritualized composition where stereotypes are called out for new service or renewed service in a conflict which itself is a remanifestation of a familiar problem."[58] This link between persona and stereotype indicates that personae may be viewed as symbolic condensations of role types that, when enacted, imply a host of preexisting narrative elements and character traits that derive from communal cultural knowledge—that is, from shared norms or *ethoi.*[59]

For some theorists, personae are forged through the particular communicative acts of the rhetor. Drawing from Walker Gibson's *Persona: A Style Study for Readers and Writers,* Paul Campbell wrote, "far from being solely a literary product, the *persona* is *'the created personality put forth in the act of communicating.'"*[60] For other writers, audiences actively construct personae. As B. L. Ware and Wil Linkugel explained, "The rhetorical *persona* is not the rhetor *qua* person but is an attributed character created by the auditor's symbolic construction (and implied assessment) of the rhetor."[61] While scientist-rhetors may indeed attempt to cultivate a particular persona, its reception depends in large part on audience willingness to recognize and affirm it. Bernard Fisher, for instance, may cast himself as a scientific revolutionary, but others get to weigh in, alter, or affirm this construction.

Most of the time, personae are cast by ensemble, depending on the mores of the day, or in the case of Datagate, on some collective sense of the scientific ethos. John Lyne and Henry Howe noted that "the *persona* of the scientific writer as a construction of the writer has received some scholarly attention"; however, "as a construction not wholly under the author's control, *persona* turns out to be an important factor in shaping the reception of scientific discourse."[62] That is, we judge scientists and their truth claims based on their personae. For example, Francesca Bordogna called scientific personae both "the normative images of the man of science" and "collective images of the scientist," and links these personae to late nineteenth-century scientific literature that discussed "the virtues, the moral sentiments, the temper, and the emotional constitution of the man of science."[63] Indeed, the persona of the scientist faces distinct constraints imposed by a collective and changing sense of the ethos of science. What happens to scientific personae when science becomes more bureaucratized and geographically dispersed? Might a proliferation of roles, and hence the corresponding personae, threaten or enhance science's place near the top of the professions? Or might these personae signify deeper anxieties about the relationship between scientists and stakeholders, between science and democracy?

To some extent, several personae of scientists already compete for legitimacy. For example, in his essay on scientific personae, Paul Campbell identified two distinct versions of an idealized persona of science, each of which attached to particular values thought to inhere in the scientific ethos: Jacob Bronowski's vision of a "clear-eyed striving, honest" persona and Theodore Roszak's vision of a "cold, withdrawn, hostile" figure.[64] Having exposed these competing personae, he analyzed them on terministic grounds, finding objectivity, predictability, and control to be three god-terms that are fundamental to science.[65] The personae of science, for Campbell, are responsible for achieving the ends represented by these communal values. They function similarly to Merton's norms. However, in the case of physician-scientists, as we shall discover in chapters 2 and 3, the available personae of scientist-rhetors become more complicated when physicians take on the mantle of science. The traditional lines of responsibility, the collective senses of duties, become blurred and confused. Personae therefore reflect "the aspirations and cultural vision of audiences from which stems the symbolic constructions of archetypal figures."[66] Mauss's connection between types of persons, or personae, their cultural roles, and broader cultural scripts is significant for understanding how personae mediate between role, individual, and culture, because personae evoke distinct narrative universes. A persona conjures up an entire storied sequence with heroes and villains, innocents and wrong-doers.

In explaining the moral lessons and characterizations that populate the narratives about principal players in this controversy, I treat persona as a constructed public role, an image that derives from broader cultural ethoi and that carries potentiality for engendering trust or mistrust, faith or disbelief in audiences in order to induce persuasion or identification. Personae correspond to stock cultural positions or roles that exist within existing narrative frameworks that encourage certain responses over others, but which then entail different possibilities in terms of assessing character for a particular case. Yet personae also emerge from the deeper sense of ethos as a dwelling place deriving from a collective set of mores and norms. To the extent that the emergence of new personae are representative of the dilemmas of a particular era, studying personae in a science-based controversy helps to illuminate some of the tensions faced by scientists as the role responds to contemporary changes and pressures.

Voice

Yet not all scientists are alike—even when they perform similar roles. The third and final concept I borrow from the rhetorical and literary lexicon, voice, refers to the particular inflections a historical person makes as she performs her role. If ethos and persona derive, in large part, from cultural mores, voice emerges through performance. As Walter Ong put it, "Voice is the foundation for rôleplaying among men."[67] Voice is related to style, to particular linguistic choices made from among the universe of possible words. In performing the persona of scientific revolutionary, for example, a particular scientist can infuse the role with his or her unique register, a personal patois that further shapes others' assessments of that persona. In one of the few explicit treatments of scientific personae to emerge from rhetorical scholarship, Kenneth Zagacki and William Keith note that direct challenges to an existing scientific paradigm (the revolutionary persona) can be made from revolutionary, conciliatory, or conservative stances.[68] Their observation underscores the role that the use of personal language choice can make in terms of the reception of arguments. In certain contexts language that is peppered with revolutionary statements and a conciliatory tonal quality will be accepted more than that which is conservatively expressed. The words scientists employ as they go about defending themselves and others in the public sphere and the specific way in which they do so thus modulate their personae. We may have, as in Fisher's case, not just a revolutionary, but a swashbuckling revolutionary. We may have, in the case of Poisson, not just a healer, but a beneficent one whose words betray abiding care for patients above all else.

As with ethos and persona, voice encompasses a dense tangle of conflicting meanings. In fact, composition scholar Peter Elbow distinguished between five different senses of voice, which range from the sounds in a text to the notion of speaking with authority. They include: "the audible voice or intonation"; the dramatic voice (or implied author of a text); a "recognizable or distinct voice"; authority; and "resonant voice or presence."[69] These divergent perspectives testify to the richness of human preoccupation with voice and its embroilment in the same debates about language and agency as ethos and persona. Is voice the authentic utterance of a person of agency or the imprint of institutional roles emanating from a body?[70] While I do not wish to diminish or negate voice's complex meanings by considering them as mere style and sound production, I generally adopt this sense of voice as the trace of an embodied rhetor's speech when analyzing the language choices of speakers and scientists. Humans possess "demonstrably unique voices"; these are used to attribute personality traits to the presumed speaker.[71] Elbow noted the oddity of our making "inferences between the voice in a text and the actual unknown, unseen historical writer behind the text—on the basis of written text alone."[72] He observed the "ingrained habit" humans have of judging the relationship between a speaker's words and the "speaker behind the words."[73] But infer we do when encountering others' voices in written and spoken words alike.

My use of the concept of voice suggests that discourse emanates from an embodied subject even when written and even while bearing the imprint of institutional and cultural constraints and possibilities. Thus it encompasses both the physical aspects involved in sound production or the commission of words to print, but it also reflects an individual style of speaking involving a set of lexical and diction choices that are characteristic of a particular person. In sum, voice illuminates the tenuous relationship between discourse, character, broader structures, and an actual, historically situated speaker. Although their personae were up for grabs in public life during Datagate, somewhere along the way actual persons—Bernard Fisher, Roger Poisson, Fran Visco, and John Dingell—drew breath and produced words. Somewhere along the way these same persons lost control of their words as these words circulated public spheres more broadly.[74] Joined by a chorus of others' assessments of these players, distinct personae emerged that were inflected by the residual traces of the voices of the historical persons. While I privilege voice as an individual stamp on language for much of this book, in chapter 4 I recover the sense of voice associated with giving agency to disempowered subjects when I analyze how breast cancer advocates participated in Datagate. They both spoke with particular voices and "gave voice to" concerns shared by their collective community.

The concepts of ethos, persona, and voice tap in to larger contemporary debates about agency and language. How much freedom does a speaker have in inventing a self through words? Ruth Amossy explains that "the idea that a discursive image of self can be influential implies that it is possible 'to do things with words,'" a view that has been challenged by postmodern scholars who deconstruct the notion of a Cartesian subject who serves as the "seat of origin" or discourse.[75] Indeed, the humanist idea that ethos is the argumentative force of a self constructed through strategic language has serious limitations according to some critical and postmodern theorists who believe that selves are not active agents that create rhetoric, but are instead resultant of larger sociohistorical and institutional forces. This view is shared by a number of postmodern thinkers, such as Pierre Bourdieu, Michel Foucault, and Jacques Derrida. Bourdieu, for example, charges that "the power of language and its ability to 'act' are not rooted in its inherent possibilities; instead, they are determined by social circumstances and power relations."[76] For Bourdieu, the force of language comes, therefore, not from ethos or persona constructed by the speaker, but from "the access he can have to the language of the institution, that is, to the official, orthodox and legitimate speech."[77] Whereas an Aristotelian view of ethos or the humanist vision of voice might overemphasize a rhetor's ability to freely choose and present a desired self, the poststructural tends to erode ethos and voice to a degree that renders rhetors largely impotent. Each perspective represents a distortion of rhetorical exchange in its own way. In my view, existing cultural forces limit the possibilities for character construction, but rhetors still operate within a field of play in terms of their linguistic choices. To complicate matters, existing conceptions of a speaker's character interact with other images of a self projected through language. Moreover, in contemporary credibility contests, the character of key players is constructed collectively through mediated processes in which various stakeholders offer testimony about the habits of other players, which are used for determining trustworthiness and reliability.[78]

To review, to speak and write of rhetorical character in science-based controversy involves enriching our understanding of the rhetorical constitution of character from a mistaken conflation with ethos to a fuller understanding of the interrelations between ethos, persona, and voice. In what follows, ethos refers to recognizable communal characteristics, the available norms or values of a group or culture. These norms circulate culture broadly, and although they are malleable through language, they are largely preexisting. Personae, or recurrent stereotyped roles, emerge from the particular features of this sense of ethos as a communal dwelling place and, in turn, constrain potentialities for evaluating the credibility of individual scientists. We may think of a persona embodying a set of activated norms, "the mask that is there before any person turns up to fill it."[79] Personae therefore mediate between communal ideals and the individual performance. Voice, by contrast, refers to a performance of role, to the particular language choices of a speaker, his or her tone or inflection. In controversies such as Datagate, the voices of speakers are often refracted through mass-mediated forms; voice thus modulates persona and challenges or affirms ethos. By detangling ethos, persona, and voice and by demonstrating their complicated links between group norms and individual performance, we come to see how, during science-based controversy, the stories we tell craft distinct but competing personae that not only draw from the inventional wellspring of the scientific ethos but also shape audience assessments of individual scientists' reputations and credibility, which are modulated by the voice of those scientists as they attempt to bolster or repair their reputations. Although this process of character construction is not specific to science-based controversies, widespread commonsense beliefs about science affect the available argumentative resources for principals trying to restore their character in cases where science and public affairs intermingle.[80] But because the particularities of each case impinge upon their progression and meanings, a fuller understanding of the contexts informing Datagate is instructive.

DATAGATE'S CONTEXTS

Ethos, persona, and voice conjoined powerfully in Datagate and were deeply intertwined with three primary sociohistorical contexts. The rise of the clinical trial as the gold standard in biomedicine, the politicization of breast cancer research and treatment, and growing awareness of the perils of research misconduct paved the way for public outcry and political involvement in the case of Poisson's falsified breast cancer data.

The Rise of the Clinical Trial in the Context of Big Science

The ascendancy of the modern clinical trial within the context of big science formed the backdrop within which Bernard Fisher would promote the randomized trial standard for his breast cancer research. The story begins just two years after Bernard Fisher completed medical school, when Vannevar Bush published his 1945 report, *Science—The Endless Frontier*. The success of science seemed all but assured, as Bush argued that public and private colleges and universities offered the "best home for basic research in medicine, science, and engineering."[81] Bush believed that locating basic research within the confines of the university rather than just in the commercial sphere would insulate science from the biased interests of business that might corrupt the pursuit of truth. Although there was considerable debate about Bush's recommendations, their adoption shifted managerial control of science away from Washington and toward scientific leaders housed in universities and colleges. Scientists received federal funding and gained autonomy provided they complied with federal regulations and assisted with national goals in areas such as defense and infrastructure.[82] "In return," notes science historian Marcel LaFollette, "scientists promised unassailable intellectual integrity, comprehensive and reliable expert review at all stages of research (the 'peer review' system for proposals and publications), and political accountability."[83] During the 1950s Cold War environment, the growth of government science agencies such as the National Science Foundation (NSF), the NIH, and the Atomic Energy Commission (AEC) would funnel money into the growing ranks of scientific and medical researchers housed in America's academic institutions. At this time, "science basked in the glory of extraordinary technological and medical achievements: life-saving new vaccines, astronauts on the moon, microminiaturization, and electronic computers. There was little scandal and, seemingly, little cause for closer attention."[84] Money continued to flow. By the fiscal year 2000, the U.S. Public Health Service (PHS) alone provided more than $12 billion of support for biomedical and behavioral research to some twenty-two hundred academic institutions across the country.[85] Laboratories grew larger and more geographically dispersed even if they contributed to a centralized mission. What might previously have taken a lone researcher a lifetime of computation and analysis could be accomplished by institutions employing hundreds of scientists marshaling ever-advancing technological prowess. Hence, conditions were ripe for both an explosion of scientific knowledge and its associated practice, and for a fraying of trust—that essential element of scientific pursuits. As an increasing number of far-flung scientists contributed to large-scale projects from around the globe, and as they became more isolated from their publics, the seeds for mistrust were quietly sown, for investigators were shielded from one another and, at times, from broader oversight.

Meanwhile, the concept of the modern clinical trial was taking hold. In some sense, *experimentation* has always been part and parcel of medical practice. Since patients do not respond uniformly to medicines and surgeries, prescribing treatment is a matter of "trial and error." Yet, since the 1865 publication of Claude Bernard's influential treatise, *An Introduction to the Study of Experimental Medicine*, systematic clinical experimentation has grown.[86] In recent years, the term *research* has been adopted by medical professionals to differentiate a "class of activities designed to develop or contribute to generalizable knowledge" and to distinguish these activities from the "experimental attitude" inherent in every clinical encounter.[87] In the 150-some years since Bernard and others advocated an experimental approach to medicine, the norms regarding medical experimentation have coalesced into a set of standards that adhere to the scientific method. Moreover, a host of protections for human research subjects initially articulated in the 1946 Nuremberg Code and later codified in the *Belmont Report* promoted an ethic of respect for human experimentation subjects. At the turn of the twentieth century, as Susan E. Lederer has shown, medical experimentation remained an idiosyncratic practice, subject to the scruples of individual scientists.[88] Some physicians experimented on themselves and their family members, while others used larger populations of disadvantaged citizens from prisons and orphanages. Although norms of scientific conduct concerning biomedical research were already beginning to coalesce at this time, it was not until 1948 that the *British Medical Journal* published the results of what is widely credited as the first modern randomized clinical trial (RCT), "Streptomycin Treatment of Pulmonary Tuberculosis."[89] The study's significance lay in the fact that it incorporated a control group and a blind randomization design so that even participating doctors did not know which patients were receiving the antibiotic streptomycin and which were in the placebo group. Bernard Fisher was five years out of medical school at the time.

Between now and then, the modern double-blind randomized clinical trial exemplified by the streptomycin trial became the foundation of medical therapy. Except in exceptional circumstances, if a new therapy has not undergone the rigors of this sort of clinical test, its safety and efficacy are not accepted. To provide suitable populations for clinical research, complex associations of cooperative, multisite research groups linked academic research institutions across the globe in the common effort of advancing the state of medical knowledge. The NSABP is an early example of this rising trend. Its first trial, initiated in 1958, garnered data from twenty-three U.S. doctors. By 2002, more than five thousand researchers—including nurses, physicians, and administrators—at two hundred institutions in the United States, Canada, Puerto Rico, and Australia participated in NSABP clinical trials.[90] But when Bernard Fisher became NSABP chair, the idea of using clinical trials to prove the efficacy of surgeries for breast cancer was rather controversial. Thus, Fisher had to persuade his colleagues that clinical trials were necessary to determine the success of surgical options for breast cancer. His colleagues were recalcitrant; Fisher therefore faced a rhetorical battle that fomented a construction of his character as swashbuckling revolutionary, a story that will unfold in chapter 3. But at the same time, he became a champion of a new form of breast cancer treatment that questioned decades of received surgical wisdom.

Challenging Halsted's Radical Mastectomy: The Science of Breast Conservation and the Rise of Patient Autonomy

Amid the rise of clinical trials in an environment of large-scale collaborative projects, the second backdrop for Datagate concerned the contentious and highly politicized history of breast cancer treatment, what renowned breast cancer physician Dr. Susan Love has called "slash, burn, and poison," short for surgery, radiation, and chemotherapy.[91] Despite the fact that both mortality from and incidence of breast cancer seem to be rising in the Western world, the scourge is an ancient one. Standard histories of the disease begin by noting that the Edwin Smith Surgical Papyrus, written in Egypt between 3000 and 2500 BC, describes "bulging tumors," believed to be the earliest known reference to breast cancer.[92] Egyptian scrolls from fifteen hundred years later prescribed treatment for breast cancer by knife and with fire.[93] Other early references to breast cancer appear in the Hippocratic corpus, which identified menopause as its cause, and first-century Roman Aulus Cornelius Celus's *De Medicinia*, which outlined four stages of the disease. Yet, throughout history, two main considerations have influenced the choice of breast cancer treatment: the extent of the disease and the prevailing theories about whether the disease was a local or systemic phenomenon. If the disease was thought to be local and confined to the breast, and if the tumor was deemed capable of being extracted, it was often surgically removed. Second-century Roman physician Claudius Galen, who believed that breast cancer was caused by an excess of black bile, for example, advocated bleeding, purging, and dietary regiments—that is, systemic therapies designed to eliminate black bile. However, even Galen called for tumor removal when the tumor appeared on the surface of the breast.

By the middle of the nineteenth century, debates persisted about whether breast cancer surgery did more harm than good; however, several innovations paved the road to the adoption of a surgical approach. In the late 1800s, laboratory experiments in Europe encouraged a local explanation of the disease. German scientist Rudolph Virchow demonstrated that in pathological tissue specimens, cancer arose from isolated clusters of diseased cells. Virchow used his observations to argue that tumors thus spread locally through the lymph nodes (rather than through the bloodstream). In his view, the lymph nodes acted as weak filters for the cancerous cells. Other scientists expanded on this work and used it to advocate for removal of not only the breast but the surrounding muscles and lymph nodes as well.[94] William Stewart Halsted, an 1877 graduate of New York's College of Physicians and Surgeons, went abroad to study European surgical techniques, as was the custom of many top-ranking graduates during this time. In Europe, Halsted, who learned of antiseptic surgery based on Pasteur's germ theory of disease, was exposed to the application of laboratory studies to clinical medicine and observed celebrated Swiss surgeon Theodor Kocher's meticulous surgical techniques, which combined careful control of bleeding with fine silk suture work.[95] Halsted also attended lectures by surgeons who advocated removal of more breast tissue than previous surgeons had spared. When he returned home, Halsted engaged in a series of laboratory studies on tissue healing and suturing before advancing the new procedures he had learned in Europe. When his studies began to suggest that the European techniques had merit, Halsted set out to refine them. In 1895 he published his first article on the subject, "The Results of Operations for the Cure of Cancer of the Breast" in the *Johns Hopkins Hospital Reports,* which reported on fifty breast cancer surgeries he had performed.[96] Halsted boasted recurrence rates as low as 6 percent, and his later refinements—including enhanced cosmetic effect, increased post-surgery arm function, and a skin graft to cover the incision—became the bedrock of breast cancer therapy.

In the early decades of the twentieth century, several historical developments encouraged widespread acceptance of Halsted's mastectomy. First, Carnegie Foundation educator Abraham Flexner issued an influential 1910 report titled *Medical Education in the United States.* Known later as simply the Flexner Report, it advocated medical school curricula steeped in physiology, biology, and chemistry based on the program that Halsted had developed at Johns Hopkins with three colleagues—gynecologist Howard Kelly, renowned physician-educator William Osler, and pathologist William Welch. Flexner traveled to all 155 medical schools in the United States and Canada promoting his model of medical education. His widespread adoption extended Halstedian principles, enhanced the credibility of work performed at Johns Hopkins (such as Halsted's mastectomies), and encouraged the triumph of the biomedical model of medicine, which favored physiological explanations of illness rather than those with more social, cultural, or psychological inflections. That patients themselves often paid for surgeries such as mastectomies led hospital administrators to encourage surgeons to perform them, which, in turn, afforded surgeons greater institutional authority. At the same time, the rise of professional surgery and the surgeons' belief in the superiority of Halsted's radical mastectomy encouraged pervasive acceptance of the procedure.

To be sure, Halsted's acceptance was not entirely monolithic. In fact, during the early part of the twentieth century, a number of surgeons expressed doubts about the need for radical and supraradical surgery, those that removed all of the "crown jewels of femininity" and additional flesh, even as more and more women unnecessarily underwent removal of ribs, ovaries, and portions of their chest wall.[97] For instance, in the 1930s Sir Geoffrey Keynes argued against the radical mastectomy. A spate of retrospective studies suggested success with no or limited therapy, leading to more questions about the wisdom of radical surgery. After World War I, interest in radiation therapy led some scientists to suggest that radiation provided possibilities for use alongside a more limited surgery. In time, though, these concerns would fade into the background as a new crop of surgeons returned home from World War II, where radical surgeries for a number of conditions seemed a battlefield necessity. With antibiotics to control postsurgical infection, these radical surgeries met with high success rates and thereby supported a cadre of "gentlemen soldiers" who believed in the merits of radical surgery, employed it in a variety of operations, and were rewarded for their efforts.[98] Surely, these surgeons recognized the limitations of their craft—they received letters from women who lost arm function after radical surgery and from the families of those who did not recover after surgery, but they also received scores of letters from patients who were grateful to be alive. Thus, for much of the twentieth century, surgeons advocated the Halsted mastectomy as the preferred treatment for breast cancer of all stages. Despite the disfigurement and pain produced by Halsted's procedure, the "classic radical mastectomy," and several modifications to it, offered several generations of women a chance at life after a breast cancer diagnosis. By mid-century the Halsted mastectomy dominated surgical practice for breast cancer, even as doubts about its necessity began to swirl.

When patients began to question physician authority in the 1970s, many would decry extensive breast surgeries as torturous barbarity. Before public awareness campaigns, annual screenings, and mammographic technology, however, it was not uncommon for women to become riddled with tumors that, left to their own devices, grew to the size of cantaloupes and larger.[99] Sarah Sim, a Nebraskan pioneer, mother, and farm wife, became afflicted with advanced breast disease in 1880. Sarah's brother John described her condition in a letter to their sister:

Sarah has been confined to bed constantly since Thanksgiving. Her right breast is enlarged to nearly the size of a lady's head and is as hard. A tumor or outgrowth from the lower right side as large as my fist and 3 smaller ones, 2 of which have opened on the upper part. Occasionally she is taken with bleeding from the larger tumors which weakens her greatly and great care is exercised in dressing the breast to prevent bleeding. She is able to lay only in one position and is only out of bed once in 24 hours . . . I have little in fact no hope of her recovery. [Sarah's husband] Sim thinks unless she improves, she cannot last to exceed 3 months.[100]

Although radical surgical intervention would not have saved Sarah's life, it would have provided some relief, and in that regard, surgeries such as the Halsted mastectomy and its variations were not as inherently barbarous as their later vilification would suggest. Put simply, in its heyday the radical mastectomy represented the best medical thinking of the time, even though it is unquestionably a massively disfiguring and debilitating procedure. The Halsted mastectomy was also a significant improvement over earlier interventions, which sometimes involved application of caustic substances, hot irons, or even amputation followed by administration of "searing heat," with results obviously more deleterious than ameliorative.[101] Nonetheless, starting in the 1970s, NSABP research helped to dislodge the dominance of Halsted's mastectomy against a tidal wave of resistance from surgeons who argued that Halsted's method worked and that surgical research was unethical.

NSABP's best-known breast cancer clinical trial, the B-06 Protocol, was particularly influential in disrupting the tenacious support for Halsted's method. The results of this study, published in 1985 and 1989 in one of the world's most widely read medical journals, the *New England Journal of Medicine,* demonstrated that breast-conserving lumpectomy with followup radiation of the breast was equally effective to the disfiguring breast-removing mastectomy for early-stage breast cancers.[102] These results, which favored breast conservation over breast removal, were hailed as a boon to women and called nothing short of a revolution in women's health care.[103]

The fact that NSABP studies of alternatives to Halsted coincided with broader cultural movements that rejected the paradigm of "surgeon knows best" helped these alternatives to achieve even greater prominence. In growing numbers women were deciding not to undergo radical surgery, as chapter 4 shall reveal. Indeed, the surge in breast cancer activism in the 1970s and the budding feminist challenges to physician paternalism transformed the doctor-knows-best model of patient care, promulgating a restructured clinical relationship in which women could be active partners in their care. Women like fifty-year-old writer Babette Rosmond resisted physicians' professional authority when they refused to accept the Halsted radical mastectomy. "I, alone, am in charge of my body," Rosmond wrote in her 1972 book, *The Invisible Worm: A Woman's Right to Choose an Alternate to Radical Surgery*.[104] Two years later, Washington, DC, journalist Rose Kushner launched her campaign to involve women in their treatment, which resulted in her partnering with Bernard Fisher to promote breast conservation. Meanwhile, Betty Rollin's *First, You Cry* and Audre Lorde's *The Cancer Journals* further pushed the boundaries of public conversation by challenging physician paternalism and openly expressing sorrow at losing a breast.[105] It was NSABP research that provided the scientific backing for these challenges. Yet, despite the excitement of the times, there were shadows on the horizon. NSABP's B-06 project happened to be the trial that informed the decisions of Jill Sigal and many other women to undergo lumpectomy, and it just happened to be one of the trials in which NSABP researcher Roger Poisson falsified data. Against the background of large-scale, multisite clinical trials and growing challenges to the breast cancer orthodoxy, the public and the scientific community attained heightened awareness of abuses that undermined trust in the system of science and threatened its autonomy and power.

Growing Responses to Research Misconduct

To be clear, data falsification in B-06 was hardly an aberration. Accordingly, the final backdrop for NSABP Datagate is increasing concern over research misconduct accompanied by bureaucratic changes aimed at staunching its spread. Starting in the 1970s, a number of well-publicized occurrences of research misconduct captured public attention. Consider, for instance, the case of William Summerlin, the Sloan-Kettering physician whose 1974 research involved grafting skin from black mice onto white ones. Summerlin's colleagues first became suspicious of his work when they noticed that the black skin grafts rubbed off when dabbed with isopropyl alcohol. When confronted, Summerlin confessed to creating the "grafts" with a black felt-tipped marker. At the time, members of the public and scientific community seemed content to dismiss Summerlin's actions as an isolated aberration that seemed to have no immediate effect on research misconduct policy. Suspicions of fraudulence in Oxford-educated Cyril Burt's published studies on the genetic contribution to intelligence also circulated during the mid- to late 1970s. Burt's publications argued that genetics, rather than being a member of the British upper class, accounted for a child's giftedness. Two years after Burt's death in 1972, Princeton University's Leon Kamin reported discrepancies in Burt's figures. Informal investigation suggested that Burt may have falsified and fabricated data and invented the existence of co-collaborators. Even his biographer, respected historian Leslie Hearnshaw, concluded publicly that Burt was "guilty" of scientific misconduct.[106] Like that of Summerlin, the Burt case was regarded as a fascinating and controversial case, though not a policy-inciting one.

Prior to the 1980s, then, research misconduct was handled in an informal and uneven way. LaFollette notes that the "tendency amongst colleagues of an accused scientist to cite deviant personality, momentary misjudgment, or external stress persisted throughout the 1970s."[107] Institutions handled allegations in-house under a veil of secrecy, as it was in their best interest that such incidents be contained. But during the early 1980s, two prominent events prompted public discussion about research misconduct policy: a particularly egregious case of research misconduct at Harvard University and the first of many congressional hearings devoted to the matter of research misconduct. In 1981 prolific publisher and rising cardiology star John R. Darsee was testing therapies for myocardial infarctions—colloquially, heart attacks—on dogs as part of an NIH-sponsored protocol. One evening, coworkers, armed with growing skepticism about Darsee's un-replicable results, observed the scientist attaching a measuring device to a dog and beginning to make tick marks at intervals of "'day one,' 'day two,' 'day three,'" making it appear as if he had collected the data over a period of several weeks. Confronted, Darsee claimed he had lost the original data and was reproducing from memory markings he had already completed according to protocol. Subsequent investigations would reveal substantial anomalies and a history of fabrication dating back to Darsee's graduate student days at Notre Dame. The prominence of Harvard, Darsee's record as a prolific publisher, and the importance of the federally funded cardiac research incited public outcry.[108]

Partially in response to this case and partially because of his concerns about recombinant-DNA research in the late 1970s, former vice president Albert Gore Jr., then a young Democratic House representative and chair of the Investigations and Oversight Subcommittee of the House Science and Technology Committee, wasted little time in calling 1981 congressional hearings on the matter of scientific integrity. Titled "Fraud in Biomedical Research," this first-ever U.S. congressional hearing on research misconduct called the heads of the NIH and the National Academy of Science (NAS) to testify on the lack of standardized procedures for handling misconduct. "At the base of our involvement in research," maintained Gore, "lies the trust of [the] American people and the integrity of the scientific exercise."[109] With these words, Gore ushered in a new era of scientist-government skirmishes over research misconduct. A year later, *New York Times* journalists William Broad and Nicholas Wade penned the best-selling *Betrayers of the Truth*, which chronicled research abuses, particularly in biomedicine.[110] Alexander Kohn's *False Prophets* followed in 1986, and before long, prominent scientists such as David Baltimore, Thereza Imanishi-Kari, Robert Gallo, William Summerlin, Herbert Needleman, Margaret Fischl, and Bernard Fisher were routinely called before Congress on research misconduct–related matters.[111] John Dingell held these hearings nearly annually between 1988 and 1994. "We do not wear lace on our drawers as we conduct our investigations," said Dingell. "I'm not paid to be a nice guy. I'm paid to look after the public interest."[112] The climate of the hearings reflected his reputation for tough-mindedness.

Against the backdrop of these hearings, a number of federal regulations and institutional policies evolved to promote probity in research. These policies, at least officially, replaced the informal ad hocery of previous decades and eventually culminated in the Office of Science and Technology Policy's (OSTP) unified federal research misconduct policy that went into effect on December 6, 2000, after an extended period of public discussion.[113] The OSTP policy marked a watershed moment in the history of U.S. treatment of deceptive research, as it was the first time that a uniform standard of misconduct would be applied to all federally supported research. Yet when the details of Datagate circulated within the public sphere, confusion about research misconduct policy abounded. One year before Datagate's publicity, the National Academy of Science's Panel on Scientific Responsibility and Conduct of Research found that the "absence of a clear, explicit definition [of research misconduct] that focuses on actions highly detrimental to the integrity of the research process has impeded the development of effective institutional oversight and government policies and procedures designed to respond to such actions."[114] Conflicting policies thus created both procedural pandemonium and possibilities for containment for administrators who were unsure of the ethical and institutional requirements in a given case. This lack of clarity was almost certainly a factor in NSABP Datagate, wherein administrators and other players invoked the confusion as a defense of their actions. Despite the muddled terrain, Datagate was thus made possible by changes in twentieth-century scientific practice ranging from the establishment of clinical trials in the context of big science, the rising challenges to breast cancer orthodoxy and physician paternalism, and a growing tide of concern about abuses to the ever-growing research process. In short, a storm was brewing, and perceptions of character comprised a central means of sorting out the confusion.

CONCLUSION: TOWARD A RHETORICAL PERSPECTIVE OF CHARACTER IN SCIENCE-BASED CONTROVERSY

My analysis turns our attention to the struggle over the character of those who participate in science-based controversies. In the chapters that follow, I am chiefly concerned with what happens to the character of scientists and other stakeholders as science-based controversies unfold and, in turn, how rhetorical constructions of the principal players transform the relationship between knowledge and character. As a rhetorician of science, I examine the consequences of language—and in this specific case, rhetorical constructions of character—in terms of the overall science-based controversy, its dynamics and meanings. In high-flying science-based controversies such as Datagate, perceptions of character act as barometers of whether or not or to what degree stakeholders accept particular scientific truth claims, thus demonstrating the connection between character and knowledge and its capacity for conversion during credibility contests.

By highlighting the rhetorical work of character construction in science-based controversies and by disentangling ethos, persona, and voice, this book offers a novel approach to understanding such controversies. According to this perspective, science-based controversies are deeply influenced by the outcomes of a collective process of character contest. Accordingly, analyzing the interrelation of ethos, persona, and voice in science-based controversy allows us to discover that our personae, in fact, reflect shared visions of the scientific endeavor. Thus, in the responses of scientists and advocates in Datagate, we are confronted with not just self-representation but a collective process of identity formation that evokes normative considerations of what a scientist ought to be, of what science ought to be. The characters that enlivened Datagate are a screen onto which we project our hopes and fantasies for science in the modern world. They are, in short, as much a reflection of our collective wishes and anxieties about biomedical science as they are about particular scientists and other key players. As we traverse the contours of Datagate in the chapters that follow, we will explore the contested characters of Roger Poisson, Bernard Fisher, and breast cancer patients, advocates, and politicians, inquiring what these characters reveal about the dilemmas of our quest for trust and truth, about science and its stakeholders, and about the overall position of science in lives that are increasingly bathed in technical knowledge and expertise.

2

A Beneficent Healer and a Career-Minded Falsifier?

Physician Researcher Role Conflict and the Janus-Faced Dr. Roger Poisson

In the fallout from the public disclosure that he had falsified North America's landmark breast cancer data, Dr. Roger Poisson became a doctor in disgrace. He was summarily shamed by the medical community, disbarred from federal research funding, and forced from his academic job. Ten months after Datagate first made headlines, the January 1995 issue of *Discover* magazine admonished readers about "yet another wayward researcher, playing fast and loose with his data," who "sullied the name of science."[1] *Discover*'s saga of Roger Poisson, alliteratively titled "Doctor Doctors Data," cast the Montreal surgeon-cum-NSABP-investigator as a deviant whose decades-long duplicity undermined more than his own reputation. "By fabricating trial data," journalist Denise Grady explained, "Roger Poisson brought down both himself and NSABP cancer trial head Bernard Fisher."[2] Although it is arguable whether it was Poisson's misdeeds or public perceptions of Fisher's reticence about them that angered patients and health-care advocates more, the discovery of Poisson's deceptive data triggered condemnation. Headlines hinting at his misconduct, the horrifying idea that a doctor had messed with something as sacred as breast cancer treatment research, sent shockwaves through the medical community, alarming medical practitioners, patients, and breast cancer advocacy groups and tipping off the hullabaloo that brought the backstage wrangling of biomedical research into public light. U.S. media attention would quickly center on Fisher, but in the meantime Roger Poisson spent an intense period in the limelight.[3]

The ensuing contest over Poisson's character exposes underlying normative tensions in biomedical research. Science studies scholar Dorothy Nelkin once observed that "controversies over science and technology reveal tensions between individual autonomy and community needs" and "reflect the ambivalent relationship between science and other social institutions such as the media, the regulatory system, and the courts."[4] *"L'Affaire Poisson,"* as Datagate became known in the Canadian media, exposed fissures between scientific autonomy; breast cancer patients' preferences; and the values of politicians, the press, and funding agencies. My analysis of Poisson's characterization in U.S. and Canadian media and international medical journal articles therefore generates instructive lessons about how the rhetorically constituted characters of science-based controversies divulge cracks in communal understandings of appropriate scientific practice. Poisson suffered expulsion from the church of science, yet recurrent characterizations of his actions raise important considerations for contemporary scientific practice and its broader relation to public life.

As this chapter details, dominant characterizations of Roger Poisson pivoted on two conflicting countenances: the personae of beneficent healer and that of an unscrupulous, career-minded research-scientist-turned-fraud. Like Janus, the two-faced god of Roman mythology associated with portals, passageways, and doorways, Poisson appeared caught between two worlds—the mythos of the ancient and humane art of healing and the contemporary rigors of clinical science. In his well-known *Science in Action,* philosopher of science Bruno Latour used a Janus analogy to differentiate between the black box of "science already made" and the open controversies of "science in the making."[5] One of Janus's faces looked to the past and the other to the future. My analogy similarly invokes Janus's bidirectional viewing: the beneficent healer peers into an idealized vision of the past where doctors' overriding concern was the individual patient, while the career-minded researcher watches the future of large-scale, bureaucratized research endeavors. Accordingly, Janus is an appropriate figure to signify competing characterizations of a man caught between disparate but interdependent worlds. My argument that Poisson's two personae and the values they signify often collide in ways that can harm clinical trial participants is not the only lesson to be drawn from the controversy, however. These two personae, these masks onto which Poisson's actions are projected, further highlight a tension that continues to haunt contemporary biomedicine, one that is further complicated by the politics driving big science: the tension between physician and researcher. In examining the personae of Roger Poisson, then, we witness how scientific characters animate and challenge randomized clinical trials, and we consider what is gained and lost in the present configuration with its stark division between science and its stakeholders, with its expectation that doctors who treat can simultaneously be doctors who study.

This chapter thus tracks the battle over the Janus-faced representations of

Poisson, the competition between two personae that accentuate the rift between research scientists and practicing physicians. In Datagate this tension is further exacerbated by Poisson's status as a surgeon, resting as it did near the top of the medical hierarchy, and his voice, which supported the ideological tenor associated with that role and, in this case, its implicit diminishment of patient autonomy. I begin by chronicling Poisson's rise through the ranks of the NSABP. I then consider how the personae of the beneficent healer and the career-minded researcher expose a fundamental and quite possibly intractable tension in the contemporary biomedical landscape. Because Poisson mounted a vigorous defense of his actions in both Canadian popular media and in international medical journals, I track his dueling characterizations across newspaper coverage and medical journal articles. I then interpret apologia produced by Poisson and his attorney against those texts responding to Poisson's rhetoric. These latter texts emphasize the persona of career-minded scientist-turned-fraud. The idea is to expose the clash between the two personae—the first emanating from Poisson and his defense, and the other cultivated largely by the medical establishment—and to analyze what this tension means for the underlying dwelling place of biomedicine and the clinical trials that sustain its influence and power in contemporary life.[6]

ROGER POISSON MOUNTS A BATTLE AGAINST MASTECTOMY

Roger Poisson was but one of several hundred health-care professionals involved in NSABP studies and one of 89 who contributed data to the much celebrated B-06 lumpectomy trial. As he advanced at the University of Montreal, his participation and leadership in NSABP studies increased. In 1965, while study director Bernard Fisher completed a Fulbright scholarship in Peru, Poisson joined the faculty at the University of Montreal as a *chargé d'enseignement*—what academics in the United States would call a lecturer. By 1980 he had worked his way to full professorship.[7] Five years earlier, Poisson had joined the NSABP clinical trials group because their upcoming B-06 study was of "great interest" to him.[8] "I was quite enthusiastic about it," he recalled in 1994, "I've been fighting total mastectomies for the last 23 years."[9] His enthusiasm produced results: he went on to enroll 19 percent of the total number of B-06 participants. All told, between 1977 and 1991, Poisson oversaw investigators at Saint-Luc Hospital in enrolling 1,511 patients into 22 NSABP trials, ranging from 354 entered into the B-06 lumpectomy trial to less than 20 patients in each of nine other trials.[10] Poisson's success thus interlaced tightly with that of the NSABP.

By most accounts, Poisson was a caring and committed surgeon with a profound interest in helping women with cancer save their breasts. When media attention forced his resignation from the University of Montreal in 1994, a colleague wrote, "During all his years of service on our faculty, he was recognized as a highly competent surgeon and a dedicated teacher."[11] Canadian journalist Fran Lowry offered a similar portrayal when she recalled a 1984 interview she conducted with Poisson when Fisher, in Canada promoting B-06 results, had banned the media from his "public" talk on the trial's results. Lowry explained, "I have conducted many interviews with many doctors over the years and can usually remember few, if any, details about them, but I remember that interview very well."[12] Lowry's reminiscences emphasized Poisson's empathy and devotion to his trade: "As we talked, Poisson never rushed me and he took plenty of time to answer all my questions. This was notable—as a rule, surgeons are always in a hurry. But what I really remember is the compassion he showed for women with breast cancer. I remember him being very concerned that they be spared the mutilation that comes with mastectomy. Why not just remove the tumour and preserve the breast—if that was possible—and then treat with radiation and perhaps chemotherapy?"[13] In Lowry's portrayal, Poisson became a humane practitioner, a rara avis among the stereotypically harried and arrogant surgical orthodoxy. This depiction accentuated his passion for breast conservation as a means of providing attentive patient care and underscored the energies he directed toward women with breast cancer. Participating in NSABP research was one way Poisson could advance his broader goal of promoting breast-sparing surgical innovation. Years later, his faith in lumpectomy would undermine his role as researcher, for it flew in the face of developing research norms, which posited that investigators should enroll patients in clinical trials only when a genuine state of uncertainty about treatment options exists. Poisson, however, positioned himself as a fighter against the agonizing but deeply entrenched breast-removing mastectomy and as a long-term advocate of breast-sparing lumpectomy.

As we witnessed in chapter 1 and will take up again in chapter 3, the idea of executing a randomized clinical trial for mastectomy challenged orthodox views about the obligations of physicians. Some surgeons expressed concern that randomized clinical trials compromised the fiduciary relationship between doctor and patient, challenging the idea that because patients entrust their lives to the care of physicians, doctors are endowed with enormous responsibility to put patients' welfare first. Some commentators alleged that physicians enrolling patients into randomized clinical trials might be "less than entirely candid with patients about what they regarded as best for them" or that assigning patients to various treatment arms "defeat[ed] individualized care."[14] One study published in the 1984 *New England Journal of Medicine* (*NEJM*) found that only 27 percent of participating surgeons claimed to have enrolled all patients who were eligible for the B-06.[15] A whopping 73 percent of these surgeons expressed concerns that the doctor-patient relationship would be affected by B-06 enrollment efforts. Others mentioned being inhibited by a perceived role conflict between doctors and physicians.[16] That so many surgeons felt uncomfortable with clinical trial enrollment, particularly in the case of a surgical breast cancer trial, reveals the suasive victory of the randomized clinical trial over the past several decades. Formerly feared for its perceived diminishment doctor-patient relations, it is now heralded as the gold standard for ethical research.[17] The controversy over Poisson's actions in B-06, then, must be understood within this context of the ascendancy of randomized clinical trials in the latter portion of the twentieth century during a time when surgeons and others became convinced that clinical trials were a necessary component of superior medical practice. Yet this perceived conflict between the researcher and the physician anticipates the dilemmas that Poisson faced in his efforts at reputational resuscitation, for it reveals the multiplicity of roles physicians can be expected to play.

For the time being, however, as he recruited subjects to B-06, Poisson appeared to be flourishing. He enjoyed a healthy practice, loyal patients, and an ever more prominent placement in the coauthor list on NSABP research publications, becoming third or fourth author on several NSABP publications of more than a dozen listed collaborators.[18] Business continued as usual until a junior researcher in Pittsburgh noted an anomaly on Poisson's charts when she confronted duplicate but slightly different records for the same patient that only hinted at a larger duplicity. The discovery would send shockwaves through the medical community—but not for a long while.

THE DISCOVERY: "LOOK, THERE ARE TWO OF THEM!"

While examining a file from Saint-Luc Hospital, where Poisson was head of cancer research, assistant Teresa Wright reportedly exclaimed, "Look! There are two of them!"[19] It seemed the file she was handling included a pair of virtually identical records for the same patient. When a clinical biostatistician named Dr. Ann Brown joined Wright, the two women scrutinized two copies of a patient record that contained one major difference: the date of the patient's surgery. One paper listed the surgery as having occurred on June 19, 1987, but according to the other it took place on June 29 of the same year. The former date would have made the woman ineligible for inclusion in the B-16 trial in which she was enrolled.[20] What purportedly baffled Wright and Brown was that both entries were typed neatly on the forms. When Brown showed the records to her supervisors, "they were equally mystified."[21] Walter Cronin, then deputy director of NSABP's Biostatistical Center, had the following (baffling and we can imagine tongue-in-cheek) response to the discrepancy: "I figured, gee, maybe there was something different about the way the folks at St. Luc's kept records . . . They were French speaking after all."[22] But nothing came of the discovery of discrepant data until September 1990, when Cronin traveled to Montreal for a routine triennial on-site data audit required by the NCI as part of their cooperative agreement of the NSABP.[23] In Montreal, Cronin found more discrepancies and several problems with consent forms.[24] Fisher and his biostatistician Carol Redmond would later report that Cronin's impression was that there had been "'no purposeful deception or deliberate falsification, but much record-changing, perhaps resulting from [the investigator's] misinterpretation of requirements.'"[25] Cronin recommended a more intensive audit of the site to "determine the extent of discrepancies in the data."[26] Investigators found that thirteen of twenty informed consent documents were signed after that date of randomization, against NSABP and federal requirements, and they located a second instance of discrepant dates for the same surgery.[27] The media would later sensationalize the case of a dead woman for whom progress reports had been filed, but Poisson insisted that these were completed without his knowledge and noted that he had fired the offending staff member.[28]

On November 14, 1990, Cronin notified Fisher and Redmond of his audit findings.[29] The two traveled to Montreal on December 7 to meet with Poisson and his co-investigator and wife, Sandra Legault-Poisson, and to inform them that a more extensive audit would follow. According to *Pittsburgh Post-Gazette* reporters Mackenzie Carpenter and Steve Twedt, Poisson "would later say that the meeting 'chagrined and saddened' him but he didn't tell Fisher at that point what he had done."[30] Between January 30 and February 1, Cronin returned to Saint-Luc Hospital with two NSABP auditors; the troika scrutinized more than one hundred patient records, including study forms, hospital charts, clinical records, and patient charts from protocol B-18. They also reviewed random samples of records from other NSABP protocols.[31] According to the ORI's final report on misconduct at Saint-Luc Hospital, these investigators noted a number of discrepancies; yet it was not until the third day of their visit that Cronin discovered definitive evidence that the Montreal investigator had deliberately falsified data when he came across two reports for a single breast cancer patient. One of the reports had a yellow sticky label attached to it that read "*vrai*," the French word for true, while the other copy had one that read "*faux*," or false. According to Carpenter and Twedt, Cronin turned to the other two auditors and said quietly, "Look at this."[32]

Fisher has said that when he was told of the falsification, he was "devastated." He would later tell the *Pittsburgh Post-Gazette*, "I had no frame of reference relative to this situation, fraud, or anything like that."[33] While still grappling with these devastating and novel events, Fisher and Redmond notified various government agencies of Poisson's actions. In their *New England Journal of Medicine* apologia, the pair summarized their version of what happened next: "These findings led us to suspend accrual privileges immediately (February 6, 1991). The project officer at the National Cancer Institute (NCI) was also notified immediately of the problem."[34] In a matter of weeks, Poisson's fate was sealed:

> On February 8, 1991, the NSABP chairman received a letter from Dr. Poisson in which he admitted having falsified data. On February 12, we [Fisher and Redmond] sent a letter to Dorothy Macfarlane, M.D., chief of Quality Assurance and Compliance at the NCI, requesting her assistance in determining what course of action we should take. We urged that "this matter be handled as rapidly as possible" because "the patients above all must receive primary consideration." The Office of Scientific Integrity (OSI) was notified of this matter by the NCI.[35]

Poisson's sixteen-year affiliation with NSABP ended quickly. He was dismissed from his position as principal investigator for NSABP studies at Saint-Luc shortly after signing his confession. Barred from research at Saint-Luc and from receiving U.S. federal funding for eight years, he was, however, allowed to continue to treat patients.[36] The new director, Dr. P.-Michel Huet, made clear that Saint-Luc assumed all responsibility for patient follow-up for more than one thousand cases with no financial support from NSABP. Saint-Luc re-randomized tamoxifen trial participants; NSABP trials resumed at Saint-Luc under Huet's direction.[37]

Since the situation was largely kept under wraps, few people were aware of the details and extent of Poisson's travails, although some Canadian colleagues knew Poisson had changed his duties at Saint-Luc. Thus, when the story finally broke in the public sphere three years later, a mixture of shock and outrage, attack and defense swept Canada and the United States. When the Datagate controversy finally erupted, study overseer Bernard Fisher faced the lion's share of media attention. On April 30, 1994, for example, the *New York Times* reported that ORI had ordered the University of Pittsburgh to consider an inquiry into NSABP studies. The seventeen-paragraph article focused almost entirely on Fisher's management of the affair, mentioning Poisson twice in one paragraph: "Last month, Dr. Fisher was ousted as administrative head of the breast cancer studies for failing to adhere to his study's guidelines in reporting and investigating data that the Canadian researcher, Dr. Roger Poisson of St. Luc Hospital in Montreal, had admitted falsifying. The Food and Drug Administration barred Dr. Poisson for life from testing experimental drugs, and he has been barred from receiving federal funds for eight years."[38]

Although U.S. media attention quickly seized on the "man in charge," Poisson's involvement touched off a period of intense disagreement that flooded the Canadian press in late March 1994. Unlike Fisher, who initially followed his lawyer's advice to stay out of the fray, Poisson quickly mounted a media defense. In the ensuing credibility contest, three primary voices spoke for Roger Poisson: the man himself, his attorney William Brock, and some of his loyal patients. Their messages consistently constructed the persona of beneficent healer acting for the greater good of his patients. However, closer inspection reveals that in mounting this defense, Poisson himself offered fodder for the second persona that is dominant in many mediated and medical journal accounts of Poisson's actions: the career-minded researcher-turned-fraud. By examining how Poisson's self-defense taps in to deeply ingrained cultural myths about doctors' beneficent duties, we can witness a tension in the underlying norms of medical practice.

POISSON'S LETTER TO *LA PRESSE* AND THE PERSONA OF BENEFICENT HEALER

Poisson's primary apologia appeared in Montreal's *La Presse* on March 30, 1994, two weeks after the initial *Chicago Tribune* report about his falsified data.[39] The twenty-five-hundred-word open letter advanced four central themes that recur in different ratios for the duration of the controversy. These included Poisson's devotion to his patients and career, his concern for patient rights, the technical insignificance of his actions, and his status as international scapegoat. The central message uniting all four themes was Poisson's enduring commitment to patient care. He repeatedly emphasized, "My one and only goal always was to provide women diagnosed with

breast cancer the best treatment available with the least possible mutilation."[40] Poisson thus positioned himself, above all, as a dedicated doctor.

First, Poisson's letter emphasized that breast cancer treatment was his
lifeblood. His closing statement that "Breast cancer is my profession, and
my profession is my life" was extracted by newspaper editors and featured as
the opening header to his letter.[41] These words testified to his abiding commitment to breast cancer; they both opened and closed his account and
were echoed elsewhere in his letter: "I devoted my entire professional life
to the diagnosis and treatment of breast cancer and the follow-up of patients with this 'cursed disease.' I devoted a great deal of energy and time to
it, and the vast majority of my patients know that well."[42] Poisson's initial
strategies for self-defense appealed to his lifelong calling as evidence for the
seriousness with which he took breast cancer treatment. He continued to
explain, saying: "Since 1975, I took part in various clinical research protocols directed by 'The National Surgical Adjuvant Breast and Bowel Project' (NSABP). I was especially motivated to do that because of the B-06
Protocol, an American study whose purpose was to prove that keeping the
breast is as effective as total mastectomy. This is a subject that always impassioned me, especially since the end of the 60s."[43] In addition to establishing his devotion to his career, this passage implicitly argued that Poisson
would have to have been a fool to threaten what he loved so dearly, for who
would knowingly endanger his life's passion? Elsewhere Poisson explicitly
raised this point, asking, "Why would someone in my position knowingly
take such enormous risks with so few precautions if I had realized that I
was committing such a crime?"[44] Had it been intentional, he continued, "I
would surely have been much more circumspect, and used a professional, or
certainly a more skilled, well-coached and sophisticated staff."[45] While attempting to appeal to professional motives, Poisson's voice bore the residual
mark of medical authority, positioning his downfall as somehow partly at-
tributable to staff ignorance, provincialism, and incompetence. It betrayed
a certain hubris hinting that his subordinates' incompetent data alterations
were partly to blame for his fall.

Despite encouraging the perception of arrogance through criticizing his
staff, Poisson's *La Presse* letter also set the stage for later arguments regarding his concern for patient rights. This move anticipated a second theme
that became increasingly prominent in Poisson's rhetoric over time: his assertion that giving women access to better health care was a motivating factor for his data alteration. "I ardently believed that a patient who had the
possibility of taking part in a protocol was treated and followed very well

and one cannot do better. It seems to me unjust to say to a woman diagnosed with breast cancer that she was not eligible to receive the best treatment available because she fell slightly outside the parameter of the 22nd
criterion, particularly when this criterion had little or no intrinsic oncological importance."[46] In addition, he noted, "While allowing these patients
to take part in the protocols, I gave them access to good care, certainly as
good [as] if not better than if they had been treated outside the protocol."[47]
"I never wanted to compromise the health of my patients or the integrity
of their care, and I still do not believe that my patients suffered from it," he
continued.[48] Poisson thus attempted to appeal to healer status; he sought to
draw from the communal ethos of medicine to suggest, in effect, that he was
a good doctor who put patients first. But in so doing, he faced a dilemma,
because the widely cited *primum non nocere* maxim of Hippocratic medicine,
"first, do no harm," appeared in conflict with the outcomes of his actions,
which by now had cast doubt on the entire system of federally funded research and, hence, ended up harming patients.[49] Poisson therefore appealed
to patient well-being at the same time he appeared to disregard it by under-
mining a clinical trial with major breast cancer treatment implications and
thereby contributing to patient anxiety. The implicit logic of "surgeon knows
best" did not resonate with citizens more broadly, for the patient autonomy
movement had made steady gains over the course of the twentieth century,
as chapter 4 will chronicle.[50] Moreover, the appeal to his healer status, I argue,
was predicated on a fundamental misreading of the medical situation facing
patients who participate in clinical research.

Poisson's vigorous insistence that he granted superior care to patients
who participated in NSABP studies evidences what Paul Applebaum and
his colleagues term the "therapeutic misconception," or the systematic "mis-
interpret[ation] of the risk/benefit ratio of participating in research."[51] According to a resounding number of bioethicists, medical historians, and legal scholars, a physician's first obligation is to provide what Charles Fried
calls "personal care."[52] This duty dovetails with long-standing medical principles of beneficence, the notion that a practitioner should act in the best
interest of the patient (*salus aegroti suprema lex*), and non-maleficence, the
value of not hurting patients, which is succinctly expressed in the Hippocratic maxim *primum non nocere.* The concept of the "healing ethos," which
for medical ethicists "is one which combines this necessary detachment
with a genuine concern for the individual patient, an attitude which requires
a degree of empathy and emotional closeness," is another way of thinking
about personal care.[53] "Only when the medical *ethos* includes a profound
respect for the individuality of each patient," ethicists Alastair Campbell,

Grant Gilbert, and Garth Jones opine, "will it serve the true purpose of medicine—the health of the patient."[54]

The problem with clinical research, then, is that it often forces providers to subsume the individual well-being of patients, the objective of personal care or the healing ethos, under the aim of producing generalizable knowledge through protocols that do not tailor medical care to the needs of particular patients. Although Applebaum and his colleagues' original concept referred to the research subject's misconception, nothing precludes healthcare providers from adopting its assumptions as well; Poisson's rhetoric of self-defense draws from the inventional wellspring of the therapeutic misconception to argue that he was acting with his patients' best interests at heart. In crafting his defense, Poisson's beneficent healer persona aims to buck the inhumane world of clinical research by acting on behalf of individual patients. Poisson himself hinted at the role conflict he felt during his clinical trial enrollment. "He described the pressures he felt in asking a patient to participate in the study," noted Lawrence Altman in the *New York Times:* "'People who are not on the front line of the battle have no idea how frustrating it can be to prepare an eligible patient for the trial, with several pep talks and a great deal of discussion, explanation for the informed consent and to convince the patient to participate and—at the last moment—to realize that the patient' is ineligible for what he perceived to be a technicality, Dr. Poisson said. 'It is a feeling of letdown and of frustration.'"[55] Here, Poisson seemed to elide the treatment "battle" with the research front.

Readers schooled in the ethics of the modern clinical trial would likely recognize that Poisson's rhetoric conflates patients with research participants.[56] Research ethicists maintain that people who participate in research must understand that the goals of clinical trials (to better science) often conflict with the needs of patients (to get better). As Charles Weijer wrote in the *British Medical Journal* in 2000, "It is widely acknowledged that physicians have a primary duty to promote their patients' welfare."[57] "When physicians become investigators," he continued, "other ends such as recruiting enough subjects and retaining them in the trial may conflict with this duty."[58] The question thus becomes: how can physicians uphold both of these duties, which, it would appear, potentially collide in randomized clinical trials? Ethicists generally offer two ways around the problem: the uncertainty principle and clinical equipoise.

The *uncertainty principle* asserts that researchers cannot ethically ask patients to participate in research unless there is genuine uncertainty about whether the current standard of care is better than the treatment being tested. Thus, it holds that physicians who believe that one treatment is superior to another cannot in good conscience enroll a patient into a randomized trial testing that treatment, since the patient might be assigned a treatment a physician believes is inferior. Of the uncertainty principle, Weijer explains, "If they [physicians] think, whether for a wise or silly reason, that they know the answer before the trial starts, they should not enter any patients."[59] However, when there is genuine indecision about which treatment is better, a physician may ethically enroll a patient into a randomized trial. The problem with this standard, for many bioethicists, is that it leaves judgment of treatment efficacy to individual physicians, so a second standard, *clinical equipoise,* based on shared knowledge, is often advanced.

Like the communal ethos, clinical equipoise relies on community standards—in this case, of treatment efficacy. Benjamin Freedman, who introduced the concept to readers of the *New England Journal of Medicine* in 1987, advanced the motivating ideal of equal balance of alternatives. Clinical equipoise refers to a general state of expert uncertainty about which treatment arm is superior. Freedman explained that "the ethics of medical practice grant no ethical or normative meaning to a treatment preference, however powerful, that is based on a hunch or anything less than evidence publicly presented and convincing to the clinical community."[60] Moreover, "persons are licensed as physicians after they demonstrate the acquisition of this professionally validated knowledge, not after they reveal a superior capacity for guessing."[61] Thus, the locus of medical judgment normatively is to reside in widely accepted professional knowledge, not the whims of individual researchers. The concept of clinical equipoise therefore asserts that researchers cannot ethically ask patients to participate in research unless there is genuine dissensus on the part of the medical community about whether the current standard of care is better than the treatment being tested.[62] "At the start of the trial," Freedman maintained, "there must be a state of clinical equipoise regarding the merits of the regimens to be tested."[63] In addition, "the trial must be designed in such a way as to make it reasonable to expect that, if it is successfully conducted, clinical equipoise will be disturbed."[64] The principle is meant to assure that patients are protected from becoming human guinea pigs subject to the personal predilections of researchers, for it establishes that there must be a reason to believe the treatment being tested is at least as beneficial as the standard of care. Theoretically, at least, clinical equipoise can make trial participation compatible with patient care, even if in practice, by asking patients to participate in clinical trials, researchers may in effect subjugate individual patient interests to the pursuit of scientific truth for the greater good. However, an interesting twist with the

B-06 protocol was that patients were *pre*randomized in order to increase enrollment.

The prerandomization innovation resulted in a sixfold increase in accrual to the B-06 study but raised ethical questions about research design and patients' ability to withdraw from the study.[65] It also tainted the "purity" of the randomized clinical trial by removing its blind aspect, because clinicians and patients knew their assigned treatment arm. Scientifically, this was problematic because it removed the blind dimension of randomized clinical trials; ethically, it was problematic because it introduced the potential for physicians who sought consent to adapt their presentation of the treatment to ensure patient enrollment. The tension between researcher and doctor is thus further accentuated in prerandomized designs. In fact, many observers have argued for inherent ethical problems with such designs.[66] For instance, regarding B-06, Judith Prestifilippo and her coauthors have asserted that "the vast majority" of commentators "said the prerandomization design was unethical because it manipulated information that caused patients to make decisions that might have differed from those they would have made with full disclosure."[67]

Poisson's apologia brought this tension between the physician and the scientist into sharp relief. This fundamental role conflict explains how, in addition to breaking public trust, Poisson's attempts to justify his actions with appeals to patient care failed so spectacularly with both the medical community and many members of lay populations. The conflict at the heart of his Janus-faced representation implies, then, that Poisson is either a paternalistic surgeon who (perhaps erroneously) *thought* he was acting in his patients' best interests or that he promoted his own interests, and possibly those of science, above those of his patients and other research participants. Poisson fought desperately to cast himself as a tireless advocate of patient access to experimental medical treatment, as primarily a beneficent healer, yet in arguing that he achieved this aim by too vigorously enrolling women into clinical trials, he undermined his own defense. As *Washington Post* writer Kathy Sawyer explained, "It is not clear what he meant; the women already were under his care and covered under the tax-financed Canadian health system."[68]

To be fair, *clinical equipoise* was not in the bioethical lexicon when Poisson began enrolling patients into B-06 in the late 1970s.[69] Moreover, the *Washington Post* noted that "in its final report on Poisson, ORI noted that until recent years, 'a certain "sloppiness" had been considered acceptable' in large clinical investigations. It suggested that Poisson had 'deluded himself' that he was in compliance."[70] *L'Affaire Poisson* therefore touched off debates about how much research ethics Poisson should have known and how precise he should have been as a scientist, particularly as trial standards were evolving over time. At the time B-06 was launched, awareness of research misconduct was growing even if particular standards were still being worked out. Even so, some in the medical community called Poisson's defense "patchy and unconvincing."[71] "You don't have to put someone in a clinical trial to give them good care," an unnamed associate of Poisson's told the *Kitchener-Waterloo (Ontario) Record*.[72] Others maintained that Poisson could have studied the women if he had noted in publications and analysis that this subset did not meet the inclusion criteria.[73] One researcher noted that by including women who were ineligible, Poisson ironically "broadened the implications of the study."[74]

Poisson's appeals to the persona of beneficent healer did not resonate widely with many journalists. Even before his *La Presse* letter, in "A Malignant Deception" the *Ottawa Citizen* condemned Poisson for committing "a terrible wrong against his patients." "Breast cancer is worse than a wounding disease of dread and pain. It is a menacing, fearful mystery. That is why the wrong done by Dr. Roger Poisson, at Montreal's St. Luc Hospital, is so despicable." The harsh condemnation from the *Ottawa Citizen* reassured readers that "in the judgment of the best experts, in Ottawa and elsewhere, the conclusion still holds: Lumpectomies with post-operative therapy can be safe and effective. As we now know, however, Poisson's contribution to this conclusion was dishonest and unreliable." "Poisson lied," announced the author, "His lies, now revealed, can only stir the fears of those who have suffered breast cancer, and those who dread it." This unsigned editorial noted that Poisson "did not just lie to his colleagues and research supervisors at the University of Pittsburgh. And not just to the U.S. Cancer Institute, which financed his research and promoted his professional celebrity. He lied to his patients. Many were never told they were subjects of research, and so never had the chance to give or refuse their informed consent. Two women were apparently enrolled in risky drug therapy despite their explicit refusal to participate." "Poisson has been disciplined, to a point," admitted the editorial, "but all that seems insufficient, unsatisfying. Whatever his motives, Poisson committed a terrible wrong against patients in his care, and betrayed the grueling struggle against breast cancer."[75] Extrapolating from the values implicit in this editorial and others like it confirms widespread acceptance of truth-telling and honesty as ethical obligations of doctors; the ethos of modern medicine demands scruples in all matters.

The values implicit in the *Ottawa Citizen* editorial additionally evidenced a sea change in patients' attitudes away from the "doctor knows best" mentality associated with the medical practice of previous eras. Barron Lerner has noted that in the 1950s and 1960s, "up to 90 percent of doctors, generally with the family's approval, preferred not to tell patients—women and men—that they had cancer."[76] By the 1990s, the patient autonomy movement had dislodged the paternalistic impulse, replacing it with calls for transparency and self-determination in medical care; the eventual dominance of autonomy as a bioethical ideal effectively put to rest the view that doctors could withhold information from patients to "protect" them from bad news.[77]

Autonomous decision-making capacity is routinely heralded as one of the most important bioethical principles of the present era, and is enacted through the values of honesty and truth-telling that are so evident in citizen responses to Poisson's defense.[78] Formally codified in major twentieth-century bioethics research statements such as the Nuremberg Code and the *Belmont Report*, the principle of autonomy extended beyond the realm of research into the sphere of patient treatment through informed consent doctrine and legislation such as the Patient Self-Determination Act of 1990.[79] A crucial corrective for the abuses of Tuskegee, Willowbrook, human radiation studies, Nazi experimental atrocities, and widespread physician paternalism, autonomy was therefore instigated to safeguard the "rights" of individuals to exercise control over their medical treatment and care. It is predicated on the assumption of an autonomous individual agent who desires to make informed decisions about his or her own medical care. Dominant bioethics discourse and practitioner philosophy thus regard autonomy as both "a medico-ethico right and a therapeutic ideal for good patient care."[80] Transformed from an ethical ideal into a procedural practice, autonomy now requires that research subjects offer voluntary and informed consent to participate in clinical trials.

Although ethicists and other commentators argue about whether informed consent is ever fully informed or voluntary, the days of doctors' actively shielding patients from distressing diagnoses with impunity have passed. The view that technical knowledge trumps lay knowledge, however, persisted, and may have been nurtured in this case by the vestiges of collective surgical dominance in the medical hierarchy. Poisson was not merely a physician; he was a surgeon. His skill with a scalpel conferred additional status and expertise, which was undermined by the manner in which he handled data. "It takes an extraordinary amount of self-confidence to wield a scalpel with skill," wrote Christine Gorman in *Time*, "but most surgeons never approach the audacity of Dr. Roger Poisson."[81]

Tapping in to the physician-researcher role tension while offering "physician-knows-best" arguments, Poisson's third claim was that he regarded his falsifications as little more than guidelines, not rigid mandates. In short, his transgressions were not *technically significant*. He emphasized that the main criteria he violated were immaterial to the trial. "The variations in question referred mainly to eligibility criteria of patients' qualifications for NSABP protocols,"[82] he began. "Some are very important," he continued, "like the diagnosis, the stage of the disease (degree of invasion), the quality of the operational act, etc."[83] However, Poisson asserted that the criteria he violated "have little or no intrinsic oncologic value."[84] For example, "47% of the variations (54 of 115) related to the criterion establishing 28 days as the maximum time between the date of the diagnosis and the admission in the protocol."[85] Poisson noted that this criterion had been altered from 28 to 56 days in later trials, a fact, he argued, that demonstrated its insignificance. The *Washington Post* offered a "typical example" of Poisson's actions, emphasizing that the NCA had later changed the eligibility requirements: "he instructed an assistant to change the reported date of a biopsy conducted on one of his breast cancer patients from Nov. 30 to Dec. 29, 1977. The false date made her eligible to participate in the landmark lumpectomy study. The true date would have disqualified her. (The scientific standards of the trial ruled out patients who delayed major surgery by more than 28 days after a biopsy showing they had cancer, though NCI itself later loosened that standard to two months.)"[86] An official of the National Cancer Institute, Dr. Dwight Kaufman, "called Dr. Poisson's comments 'farcical,' maintaining that Poisson had no understanding or respect for the scientific method."[87]

Poisson's self-defense and its discussion in newspapers and magazines introduced technical reasoning into a public sphere that was largely ill-versed in the rules of such reasoning. Latour has explained that "when [science] controversies flare up, the literature becomes technical."[88] For Latour, during these flare-ups, rhetoric becomes "still more important" as "debates are so exacerbated that they become scientific and technical."[89] Ironically, Poisson's appeal to technical reason bolstered his self-portrayal as a healer who sided with patients against the medical establishment that offered poor treatment and breast mutilation. As a surgeon skilled in technical reasoning, Poisson implicitly asked patients and the public to accept his word—that is, to trust that this criterion had no impact on the outcome of the trial, and that his falsification stemmed from beneficence, from a greater duty to help patients. He implored them to understand his actions on the grounds that he held his patients' best interests at heart. The problem with this construction, with Poisson's persona of beneficent healer, is that it contained more than a whiff of what the contemporary autonomy movement in bioethics has labeled physician paternalism. It said, *Trust me, I know best.* Moreover, the beneficent healer construction provided fodder for members of the medical community to chastise Poisson for bucking their communal ethos. One colleague dismissed Poisson's defense of his actions, noting, "This was not sloppiness. It was real cunning fabrication."[90] The *New York Times*'s physician-journalist Lawrence Altman seized on the conundrum facing Poisson in terms of his role conflict: "Yet the reply that Dr. Poisson made to accusations . . . creates the impression of an emotionally charged researcher who deliberately ignored what he saw as trivial rules of the study more than a dispassionate scientist who strove for objectivity and precision."[91] By displaying emotion, losing sight of impartiality, and flaunting the widely shared rules of the scientific community, Poisson could thus be readily expunged from the halls of science. And he resoundingly was.

A final argument that became increasingly prominent in Poisson's self-characterization concerned his claim that he was the victim of international scapegoating. This theme had its seeds in an article that appeared just two days before his *La Presse* apologia. A March 28 *Maclean's* feature reported that "a disgraced doctor hints at a conspiracy." "Baring his wounds," the article continued, "Dr. Roger Poisson finally emerged into public view last week." Poisson is characterized as a "Montreal oncologist, who three weeks ago provoked a continent-wide scandal for falsifying data in major breast cancer studies." He "looked frail," "gaunt," and told the audience "I've been sick . . . probably as a result of the stress I've suffered." Just as reporters commented on Fisher's gravelly or tremulous voice, *Maclean's* noted Poisson's "voice quavering" as a means of humanizing the doctor's strain, yet *Maclean's* also fueled a perception of arrogant paternalism. The article revealed that Poisson "admitted that many of the charges leveled against him contained a measure of truth," yet "stoutly maintained that he was guilty of nothing more than 'too much enthusiasm' for his patients' welfare." Here, the defiant voice ascended above the quavering one. Finally, the article amplified the charge of international scapegoating. "He hinted darkly," wrote reporter Barry Came, "that his disgrace had been engineered by unnamed forces in U.S. medical and political circles." "Someone wants my skin," Came quoted Poisson. "The Montreal doctor portrayed himself as the victim of a conspiracy," Came explained, "launched by U.S. interests out to discredit both him and Canada's medical system." Came emphasized that Poisson offered no proof of the conspiracy, thereby suggesting the flimsiness of this idea, but quoted the doctor as identifying his persecutors: "'They are American senators who, rightly or wrongly, find that there is too much research money that goes outside the United States. Other senators think, rightly or wrongly, that too much American money goes to clinical research. And there is also the American surgery lobby, which is very strong. You draw your own conclusions.'"[92]

Media amplification of Poisson's *La Presse* letter furthered the theme of international competition, picking up on Poisson's claim that Quebec led North America in its use of lumpectomy over mastectomy. The following day, United Press International reported, "The former chief of oncology at Montreal's St. Luc's Hospital suggested he was targeted by U.S legislators who want to reduce the amount of U.S. research money being spent outside the country and by U.S. surgeons who opposed the study's findings."[93] Thus, Poisson dramatically attempted to rescript the story as one of international antagonism and backstabbing. Poisson repeatedly invoked this theme in subsequent interviews appearing in both Canadian medical journals and international newspapers.[94] While the idea that U.S. and Canadian scientists competed over surgical dominance might have resonated with widespread cultural stereotypes about tensions between the two nations, the "conspiratorial" flavor of these arguments also lent credence to the suggestion that Poisson was guided more by emotion than reason, which supplied further ammunition to the critics who could cast him as passionate and therefore nonscientific.

News media ventilated Poisson's four arguments more broadly in both the United States, where he received significantly less attention than Fisher, and in Canada. First, news media emphasized Poisson's dedication to his craft. For example, the *New York Times* reported that Poisson stated his goal for thirty years of practice had been to provide "the best treatment available with the least amount of mutilation possible."[95] Second, the media echoed Poisson's continual reassertion of his motive of patient beneficence. The *New York Times'* coverage of Poisson's *La Presse* letter noted that Poisson "asked not to be judged on the discrepancies in his research data but on his larger contributions to patient well-being."[96] "'Perhaps I didn't have the guts to say no to a woman," Poisson told United Press International (UPI), "but she would have gotten lower quality treatment elsewhere,'" he said.[97] The day after his *La Presse* letter, UPI reported that "Dr. Roger Poisson admitted at a press conference he gave false data during the study, but claimed it was in the best interests of his patients." Amplifying *La Presse* themes, the report noted that "Poisson said he lied about some patients' diagnosis dates in order to help women get better treatment and called the discrepancies 'insignificant." In addition, "He said in some cases a woman might have met most, but not all, of the criteria, and wouldn't have been allowed [to] enroll in the program." Poisson's lawyer, William Brock of Montreal, insisted in an interview with the *Times* that "at no time did he receive any personal benefit—that was not his motivation."[98] On March 31 Poisson granted an interview to the *Montreal Gazette*; the paper framed his discourse in terms of Poisson's "lashing out at critics": "he didn't apologize for sparking an international research-fraud scandal that has thrown into question the conclusions of major breast cancer studies. Instead, he defended his decision to falsify the records of 99 of his patients, arguing he did it for their own good."[99] Similarly, the *New York Times* repeated that by "falsifying details, he 'opened the door to better treatment, including experimental drugs,' he said."[100]

Third, print news media ventriloquized his argument of technical insignificance. "Dr. Poisson said his irregularities were of a technical nature," declared Clyde Farnsworth in the *New York Times*.[101] "He said he did it," explained the *Montreal Gazette*, "because he was frustrated by the studies' arbitrary eligibility rules that, for example, barred a woman if more than 28 days had passed since she was diagnosed with breast cancer."[102] Finally, these sources furthered the theme of international competition. The UPI report explained, "The former chief of oncology at Montreal's St. Luc's Hospital suggested he was targeted by U.S legislators who want to reduce the amount of U.S. research money being spent outside the country and by U.S. surgeons who opposed the study's findings."[103] According to the *Times*, "Poisson said that Quebec had the lowest rate of mastectomies in all of North America, one of the highest rates of chemotherapy in place of surgery, and one of the best records of early detection of breast cancer tumors in the world."[104] This theme became increasingly prominent in Poisson's rhetoric and to some extent was supported through an unlikely source: discourse in the *Canadian Medical Association Journal* (*CMAJ*), as the subsequent section of this chapter shall reveal. However, Poisson latched on to this defense so strongly that he featured it in *Le Cancer Du Sein: S. V. P. Ne Pas Mutiler* (Breast Cancer Please Do Not Mutilate), his 1994 book about breast cancer treatment, which reiterated argumentative themes of his *La Presse* letter, particularly hammering on his devotion to patients and his career. In the epilogue, titled "*L'Affaire Poisson*," Poisson met the charges directed against him in a point-by-point response. He began by noting: "The public certainly deserves more information on all this business. I devoted all of my professional life to the diagnosis and to the treatment of the breast cancer and the follow-up of the patients plagued by this 'cursed malady.' I devoted much energy and time to it, as the vast majority of my patients well know."[105] The scolding tone of his voice in this passage and the invocation of his patients as allies in his cause lacked *eunoia*, or goodwill, for audiences more generally and signifies how his surgical voice imperiously undercut assessments of his credibility. It sounded sour and defensive, thus encouraging a general suspicion of his motives.

Amplifying the theme of persecution, Poisson closed his book with a French translation of Rudyard Kipling's "If," focusing on a character who must withstand, among other indignities, professional condemnation. This 1895 poem was inspired by the tale of Dr. Leander Starr Jameson, who led about five hundred of his fellow Brits in a difficult raid against the Boers in southern Africa. It narrates the story of grace in the face of professional despair, a tale of winning even in defeat, that emphasizes trusting yourself when others do not, refusing to lie when others are lying about you, and not hating when others hate you. If you can keep your wits about you when tested, "Yours is the Earth and everything that's in it / And—which is more—you'll be a Man, my son!"[106] In invoking grace in the face of international battle, the poem enthymematically suggested the rightness of Poisson's actions, positioned the doctor as ultimately heroic in a larger struggle, and ultimately cast him as a temporary victim of forces larger than himself. It therefore encapsulated all four of the arguments Poisson used to explain his actions.

The four dominant arguments that attempted to explain Poisson's misdeeds cemented the Janus-faced characterization of Roger Poisson. Was he a beneficent healer peering toward medicine's mythical past who put his patients' interests above all else, as he and his lawyer tried so tirelessly to assert? Or was he, as many of his colleagues implied, a selfish, bumbling, career-minded researcher-turned-fraud who blatantly disregarded both his patients' welfare and the community of science? Poisson's efforts at self-construction as beneficent healer contained inventional resources for others to advance the persona of the career-minded researcher-turned-fraud, because they betrayed the trace of paternalism and pride. As the controversy progressed, Poisson attempted to shift the frame to one of international rivalry, in which he, although still the beneficent healer, fell victim to international competition and scapegoating. This move, as we shall see, did not further his cause. Indeed, once celebrated for his rising status within the cutting-edge breast cancer group, Poisson found himself vigorously excommunicated. The *Washington Post* reported that Poisson had "no known defenders in the medical community."[107] After he exposed the flaws of science, the scientific community had little room for the likes of Poisson.

CMAJ COVERAGE AND THE RHETORIC OF
INTERNATIONAL SCAPEGOATING AND COMPETITION

Because *L'Affaire Poisson* involved one of its countrymen, the *Canadian Medical Association Journal* provided a forum for members to air their concerns about the controversy. In *CMAJ*'s September 15, 1995, issue, editors presented a two-part treatment of the B-06 controversy. The first part featured an editorial focusing on research misconduct related to published articles in general. "Scientists are people, and people make mistakes," began the *CMAJ* special report "Science and Scandal: What Can Be Done about Research Misconduct." "Science corrects for their failings in the long run, although the short run is a different matter. But even this isn't the problem it once was and, paradoxically, a recent scandal may help," the report continued. After a two-sentence paragraph explaining the events following the *New England Journal of Medicine* and the public's discovery of the false data in NSABP trials, the essay outlined Poisson's career, culminating in a tribute proffered by one of Poisson's colleagues: "During all his years of service on our faculty, he was recognized as a highly competent surgeon and a dedicated teacher." *CMAJ* included noticeably less of the finger-pointing and attribution of blame found in the *NEJM,* where, as will be explored in chapter 3, dominant arguments affixed responsibility primarily on Fisher. Instead, the editors acknowledged that in research a variety of ethical quandaries inevitably arise and that humans, being humans, will make mistakes—or even deliberately buck the system. Improvements should therefore be made to the overall system. The *CMAJ* editorial observed that "virtually every editor has seen situations in which authors have exaggerated the claims of their research" and enumerated a variety of unethical research practices that a journal editor might encounter, ending with research misconduct. The ultimate recommendation: "perhaps changing the system and encouraging greater awareness will help [dishonest researchers] resist some of the temptations that lead to research fraud."[108] There is a striking contrast between these calls for systemic changes focusing on education and prevention and the establishment in the United States of a clinical trial monitoring branch and enforcement of more stringent requirements for data monitoring. Clearly, the tension between science viewed as a self-governing unit versus science seen as a publicly regulated social good lurked behind much of the brouhaha over B-06.

Reminiscences by Toronto freelance writer Fran Lowry opened the *CMAJ* interview with Poisson that followed "Science and Scandal."[109] Lowry reprinted sections of an interview she conducted with Poisson before the controversy and fragments of a new one she had after it. Lowry, obviously a Poisson supporter, fondly recalled the concern Poisson had previously demonstrated that women "be spared the mutilation that comes with mastectomy."[110] "Why not just remove the tumour and preserve the breast—if that was possible—and then treat with radiation and perhaps chemotherapy?" she recalled him asking.[111] Then, in a piece that interspersed his own words with Lowry's sympathetic summary, Poisson's voice framed the controversy as a contest between himself and two powerful enemies: aggressive and intransigent American physicians who preferred invasive procedures to lumpectomy and breast cancer itself. This is an interesting move, as it attempted to reframe the controversy from a case of fraud, the dominant frame in U.S. media and journalistic accounts, to a schism over treatment between powerful national factions, the framing that was anticipated but not fully elaborated in Poisson's *La Presse* apologia. The *NEJM* correspondence, by contrast to *CMAJ*, featured scientists' (save Poisson's) claims to have acted within the norms of legitimate science when faced with the threats posed to it by Poisson. But Poisson attempted to shift the grounds of the debate to the topics of patient care and international competition, and one might be tempted to ask whether American silence on these issues represents a concession or a resounding dismissal of their legitimacy.

In *CMAJ* Poisson maintained that he had "*appris sa leçon à la dure*"—that is, he had learned his lesson the hard way. He nonetheless speculated that the fervor behind what he believed was U.S. persecution stemmed from the U.S. medical establishment's disapprobation of his long-term advocacy of lumpectomy—a procedure that he said thwarted the preferred therapy of the U.S. medical academy. Poisson argued that Canada was superior to the United States with regard to breast cancer therapy. Whereas Canada had employed lumpectomy for a quarter of a century, the United States was still advocating use of the Halsted method as late as 1987—two years after the B-06 trial showed it unnecessary for early-stage breast cancers. "We've [the Canadians] been treating with lumpectomy for 25 years now, so it's nothing new," he observed, "yet, here you have all these Americans debating whether mastectomy still has a place."[112] Poisson invoked the cases of Nancy Reagan, Happy Rockefeller, and Betty Ford, all of whom had radical mastectomies, as evidence for the United States' intransigence regarding lumpectomies. "For some strange reason, the U.S. is behind," Poisson argued, "not only [do they have] a penchant for doing total mastectomies, but [they] also [fail to do] needle biopsies. Many old-fashioned surgeons still do old-fashioned surgical biopsies."[113] Thus, by casting himself as a scapegoat in an international battle over breast cancer therapies, Poisson attempted to revive his reputation, recasting himself as a champion of superior medical care.

The rhetoric of international competition and scapegoating reverberated through other sources. The *New York Times* reported that the sixty-two-year-old, who had been hospitalized with a "stress-related ailment" for ten days at the end of March, met with reporters alongside his attorney William Brock. According to the *Times,* "the doctor said that he had antagonized the United States medical establishment by advocating a lumpectomy rather than a mastectomy in treating breast cancer before a lumpectomy, a less disfiguring operation, became accepted practice. The establishment was now using him as a scapegoat, he said."[114] Poisson "berated his critics," reported the *New York Times,* "chiefly in the United States, who he said wanted him to blindly obey rigid research guidelines. He accused critics of persecuting him and 'taking the same attitude towards me as the States has against Somalia and Vietnam.'"[115]

Poisson repeatedly emphasized that his primary concern was the welfare of his patients. The tension inherent in the role of physician-investigator is an appeal that, except for a brief mention in Poisson's letter to *NEJM,* is surprisingly missing from most U.S. correspondence.[116] After underscoring that the dates he altered did not affect the outcome of the case, Poisson argued that he enrolled ineligible women in the trial for two primary reasons. First, he did it because he felt that the rules governing clinical protocols were to be understood as guidelines and not rigid mandates, and, second, because he believed the women he enrolled in the trial received health care and access to therapies that were superior to that of those who were not enrolled in the trial. Poisson thus attempted to rationalize his actions by appealing to beneficence: he enrolled ineligible women in the trial so that they could receive the best possible health care. As early as February 1991, Poisson wrote in a letter to the NSABP that he was not ashamed of "having done my best to enter as many patients as possible" into the trial.[117] In his 1994 *NEJM* correspondence he wrote, "For me, it was difficult to tell a woman with breast cancer that she was ineligible to receive the best available treatment because she did not meet one criterion out of 22, when I knew this criterion had little or no intrinsic oncologic importance."[118] This issue of patient rights with regard to experimental treatment versus clinical trial eligibility requirements is one that was largely muted in *NEJM* discourse. In the way coverage of this case played out in the United States, much opportunity for reflection on the modern clinical trial was forestalled.

The contest over Poisson's character is merely a small battle in the broader struggle concerning medical authority and patient autonomy within the larger context of clinical research. Poisson attempted to secure medical authority at a time when it had already eroded. Because he had both violated the code of silence of the medical profession and exposed its backstage dealings to public scrutiny, Poisson made an easy scapegoat. "Montreal surgeon Roger Poisson was apparently able to get away with years of falsifying research data on breast cancer," reports one newspaper, "because, as one medical colleague said, physicians 'aren't naturally whistle-blowers.'"[119] By synechdochic extension, Poisson's actions potentially taint his entire profession. It is little wonder that he was so vigorously excised by colleagues. Randy Allen Harris writes that "to be identifiable to a member of a group, then, is (as rhetor) to draw on its vocabulary, to echo its enthymemes, to wallow in its stylistic proclivities; in short, to evoke and perpetuate its *ethos*."[120] While Poisson may have attempted to draw on the patois of his profession, he also revealed its underbelly. As one newspaper explained, "The medical system in which they [women patients] have placed their confidence—and their hopes of a cure—has consistently put their interests behind such things as professional solidarity and institutional secrecy."[121] Although this insularity may have protected Poisson from his initial public outing, once he was exposed, excision began. Thus, the medical community engaged in a vigorous rhetoric of expulsion of Poisson even as news of other NSABP researchers engaging in similar practices surged through the press. When the community of science spoke, it censured Poisson.

WHO FRAMED ROGER POISSON? FURTHERING THE PERSONA OF CAREER-MINDED RESEARCHER AND THE RHETORIC OF FRAUD

"He was always so proud of all the patients he had on clinical trials, of what a big contributor he was and how his name was on the academic papers," claimed one of Poisson's colleagues in the *Record*.[122] By contrast to Poisson's stated motivations of patient beneficence and access to "experimental" treatments—treatments he would later assert Canadians knew were superior—medical commentators frequently cited career aspirations and professional notoriety, thereby crafting the persona of career-minded researcher-turned-fraud. Dr. Jacques Jolivet, an oncologist from Montreal's Notre Dame Hospital, noted, "Poisson's a proud man—proud to say that he puts most of his patients in trials, proud to get grants, proud to get his name on research papers. It was a long ego trip. He just lost it at one point and wound up twisting the data."[123] Lawrence Altman of the *New York Times* echoed the portrayal of Poisson's selfish motives by noting that "being a principal investigator in an important study involving a major public health problem can be a mark of distinction, even if it does not lead to financial gain."[124] While the persona of career-minded researcher-turned-fraud was emphasized repeatedly by colleagues who added their own shadings of pride and ambition to the mix, Poisson himself unwittingly contributed to the construction of this persona by frequently referring to his enthusiasm for clinical research.

However, the rhetoric of fraud itself also bolstered this persona. The discourse of fraud pervades accounts in both the medical community and the popular press, but it is not without consequence. Elsewhere, I have written how the dominant media frame of fraud in science-based research misconduct controversies serves as symbolic shorthand for a spectrum of potential research misconduct abuses, some of which rise to the level of legal fraud but many of which do not.[125] The rhetoric of Poisson's fraud is evident from Crewdson's initial headline, "Fraud in Breast Cancer Study: Doctor Lied on Data for Decade," to congressional testimony such as Jill Sigal's "anger and outrage that a doctor could possibly engage in such gross scientific fraud," to the *New England Journal of Medicine*'s repetition of articles on Poisson's fraud.[126] To a large extent, Crewdson's initial framing of the data alterations as "fraud" persisted. On March 15, two days after Crewdson's first story, the *Washington Post* article "Experts Try to Allay Cancer Fraud Fears" repeatedly emphasized "the fraud."[127] Of major newspapers that covered the story, the *New York Times* most consistently avoided the "fraud" label, instead using the terms "flawed data," "fabrication," and "falsification."[128] Michael Zerbe, Amanda Young, and Edwin Nagelhout's study of the B-06 controversy argues that "public discourse that dealt with [the B-06 controversy] focused on sensationalizing the fraud."[129] Headlines such as "Flawed Cancer Study Haunts Many Women" and "Research Fraud Breaks Chain of Trust," coupled with statements of concern by medical researchers and politicians, reinforced the message that Poisson had cheated the medical community.[130]

The argumentative effect of emphasizing fraud is to affix responsibility on perpetrators of the misconduct and on those who did not disclose it to the public. Thus, this representation drew attention to the person committing the action and left the overall clinical trial structure, inclusion rules, and the separation between science and its stakeholders unquestioned. It expunged individuals who did not conform to the seemingly fixed norms of the system. Moreover, fraud generally refers to deception for personal gain but also has a technical legal sense of deliberate deception in order to damage someone else. Thus, the term *fraud* found throughout the newspaper coverage, congressional testimony, and by the editors of *NEJM* comports more with a colloquial sense of the term than a technical one. Indeed, the *New York Times* eventually clarified its coverage of the case, noting that "because of an editing error, a front-page article on Monday about a Federal investigation of a study of breast cancer treatments referred incorrectly in some copies to the extent of wrongdoing found. Data were falsified, but there was no finding of fraud."[131] Although the legal sense may apply in this case to the extent that Roger Poisson could be seen to have altered data in order to further his career and received monetary gain via grants for doing so, his reasons for enrolling ineligible women in the trial appear more complicated than personal gain, as the forthcoming section of this chapter shall demonstrate. In short, the rhetoric promoted a facile understanding about the nature of Poisson's actions and the complexity of clinical trial inclusion rules.

Drawing from the ORI's *Final Investigation Report* on Roger Poisson, my interpretation of the six discrepancies in Poisson's B-06 data suggests that in two cases in 1977 Poisson altered the date of diagnosis—that is, the biopsy date—to make patients appear eligible to participate in the trial.[132] Two years later, he omitted a biopsy date from an ineligible patient, a practice he repeated in 1981 and 1982. Finally, in 1982 he changed a date by ten days to make a patient eligible to participate in the trial. Therefore, his misdeeds in the B-06 trial consisted of altering or omitting six dates from patient records sporadically over the course of five years.[133] Poisson's stated reasons for this practice were to allow ineligible women into the trial, which would grant them access to medical care. While many people agree that these actions constituted an affront to scientific integrity, what counts as research misconduct is sometimes a "gray area" subject to ambiguity, negotiation, and interpretation.[134] Thus, the B-06 controversy presented an opportunity for more careful public reflection about scientific practices, clinical trial enrollment criteria, and access to both health care and experimental treatments. However, in the accounts of science to emerge as the controversy unfolded, the opportunity to examine the underlying assumptions of clinical research that supported these practices largely passed without reflection. This occurred, I argue, largely because the dominant representations of scientific practice that emerged focused on individual transgressors, like Fisher and Poisson, who were framed as polluting an otherwise pure scientific practice.

A year after the B-06 controversy went public, the opportunity for more nuanced reflection occurred when Canadian physician Charles Weijer published a *CMAJ* editorial arguing, like so many others before him, that Poisson's justification of his misconduct was unacceptable. "The three claims put forward by Dr. Roger Poisson to rationalize his enrollment of ineligible subjects in clinical trials do not justify research fraud."[135] Moreover, "certain lessons for the conduct of clinical research can be learned from the affair."[136] For Weijer, the lessons of *L'Affaire Poisson* included the fact that experimental therapies should be made available to patients who are technically ineligible if no other therapies exist for their condition, each eligibility criterion should be rigorously justified, and research should be conducted to investigate the benefits of clinical trial participation. Weijer thus analyzed what the controversy suggested about clinical trials in general. *NEJM* discourse, on the other hand, did not discuss these issues, thereby missing the opportunity for critical reflection outside of the individual transgression/pollution of science model.

By contrast to the rhetoric of fraud and its corresponding persona of the career-minded researcher-turned-fraud, Poisson cast his actions in terms of harmless "white lies," an analogy that many breast cancer patients found difficult to accept. "At one point in the interview," noted the *Montreal Gazette,* "Poisson appeared to compare his data falsification to a white lie he once told about his sons."[137] Poisson reportedly said, "I did change once the birthdates of my sons in order that they be able to enroll in a tennis course. Now that's a crime."[138] The slightly surly, defiant, and unapologetic voice emerging from these accounts therefore echoed the reluctant apologist persona of Bernard Fisher, which we will encounter in chapter 3. Both men, it seems, advanced self-portrayals in which they had little to apologize for. Bolstered by their arguments of harm to self incurred by loss of reputation and vigorous assertions that their actions did not alter trial outcomes, audience attributions of medical paternalism and arrogance were confirmed to the detriment of both men's reputations and careers.

CONCLUSION: DUELING COUNTENANCES OF BIOMEDICINE

The contest to frame Roger Poisson as, on the one hand, beneficent healer, champion of women's health, and advocate of patient rights, and on the other hand, as career-minded researcher and scientific fraud taps in to deeper debates about the shifting locus of medical authority in Western society and exposes inherent contradictions between the roles of physician and biomedical researcher. In this credibility contest, the communal dwelling place of science is exposed to the harsh light of public scrutiny; because of widely shared normative expectations of scientific purity and objectivity, it falls short. Poisson's conflicting countenances therefore signify the shifting face of medicine from its mythos as a healing art to its status as a biomedical science. Like Janus, representations of Poisson signal a transition toward the future of biomedicine wherein the science of clinical trials reigns supreme.

When Poisson began participation in B-06, debates about whether it was appropriate for clinicians to enroll patients in clinical trials persisted. Fifteen years later, the ascendancy of the modern-day clinical trial was complete. To the extent that personae reflect "the aspirations and cultural vision of audiences from which stems the symbolic constructions of archetypal figures," the beneficent healer and the clinical scientist thus are found to be at odds, despite arguments that equipoise alleviates them.[139] The gap between Poisson's two personae further reveals a fundamental conflict that has yet to be completely resolved: to what extent are publics entitled to participate in facets of medical experimentation that affect their health and well-being? Despite consistent arguments for shared scientific governance, strong norms for notifying trial participants of the outcomes of research—much less problems with the data—did not emerge from this scandal or other similar controversies. Thus, the tension between physician-researcher silence and public disclosure recurs in science-based controversy; this recurrence suggests a need for broader reflection about how clinical trial participation can be structured in ways that secure participation of affected stakeholders. The issue of stakeholder participation in clinical trials comes into play even more powerfully in chapter 4, where we will explore what the characterizations of politicians and patients during Datagate suggest about the role of character in science-based controversy and their potential for promoting more democratic forms of scientific governance. However, we must first examine Fisher's characterizations in light of what we have learned about Poisson in order to gain a more complete understanding of the dwelling place of science when it intersects with public interests and political agendas.

3

The Rise, Fall, and Resurrection of a Scientific Revolutionary

Competing Characterizations of Dr. Bernard Fisher

On the morning of October 27, 2000, Dr. Bernard Fisher stood before a lectern in lecture rooms 5 and 6 of the University of Pittsburgh's Scaife Hall. Just moments before, School of Medicine dean Dr. Arthur Levine had lauded Fisher as "one of the most influential scientists of our time." Pronouncing the occasion a "once in a lifetime experience," Levine told the assembled audience, scattered about the large auditorium in a sea of white coats, blue-green scrubs, and blazers, that they would "hear firsthand from one of the handful of individuals whose work in our own lifetimes has led to a paradigm shift in the way the human body is understood and to the way in which medicine is practiced." Levine announced a list of Fisher's awards—the American Cancer Society's Medal of Honor, the American Surgical Association's Medallion for Scientific Achievement, and so on—mentioning the "millions of women worldwide who had been affected" by research conducted under Fisher's direction.[1] Fisher's return to Scaife Hall to deliver an invited "Legacy Laureate" address symbolically marked his reunification with his alma mater after his forced departure during the height of the Datagate scandal in 1994.[2] It publicly reinforced his reputation as a scientific revolutionary—one of the most enduring and, as we shall see later in this chapter, ultimately misleading scientific personae of our time.[3]

Having chronicled the contested characterizations of Roger Poisson in chapter 2, this chapter unravels the struggle to define Fisher's character in the wake of the Datagate scandal. Because of his iconic stature in the realm of cancer research, local and national newspaper coverage quickly seized on Fisher, and the *Cancer Letter* featured frequent updates on the man and his fate. The intense scrutiny of Fisher was justified, implied *Health Facts*, because "Dr. Fisher is held more accountable than Dr. Poisson."[4] In short order, the farrago of incidents and allegations that churned this controversy cohered into narrative form starring the character of science in general and the competing personae of Bernard Fisher in particular, rendering the integrity, trustworthiness, and very character of Fisher a predominant concern. Was he an overburdened researcher unwittingly caught in the crossfire of political battles beyond his control? Was he an arrogant administrator who imagined himself above scrutiny? Was he a "hero among us," as representatives from the pharmaceutical giant Zeneca would later suggest?[5] Was he a visionary so infatuated with the big picture that he forgot to oversee the everyday operations of his organization? Was he the victim of an overly zealous and unfair political campaign lobbed against big-name scientists? Fisher's rhetorical performance as Legacy Laureate suggested the latter and thus signified a transformation from vilification to vindication, a dramatic reversal of the situation six years earlier when newspaper articles reported that Fisher had tumbled from stunning heights.[6]

The preoccupation with Fisher that marked the height of Datagate raises several questions concerning the rhetorical dynamics of science-based controversies. What factors encouraged the focus on Fisher's character, and how did political contests over big science shape this frame? What were Fisher's dominant personae, how were they scripted, and by whom? Was the focus on Fisher justified? And how did these personae influence the dynamics of the controversy and its outcomes? This chapter explores these questions by charting how Fisher's competing personae vied for legitimacy in professional, political, and public spheres, and by considering what these personae mean in terms of the status of scientific knowledge and thus, in Datagate, for the fate of breast cancer patients. In contrast to Roger Poisson's dichotomous characterization as beneficent healer or career-minded fraud, conflicting countenances of Fisher abounded and revealed deeper tensions with scientific administration. I argue that three personae—the scientific revolutionary, the beleaguered bureaucrat, and the reluctant apologist—competed for credence in the initial weeks of the Datagate controversy and were eventually supplanted by a fourth, the portrait of a tragic-hero-turned-vindicated-visionary. When viewed as a whole, these personae implicitly endorsed policy outcomes that were focused on purging science of individual transgressors while obscuring broader systemic reforms that could have more substantively addressed the concerns of patients and advocates.

Because existing public narrations of Fisher's life and character provided the backdrop for reworked constructions of his character in light of allegations of scientific mismanagement, I begin by charting Fisher's role in breast cancer research and his work for the NSABP, reassembling published accounts of Fisher's life and career, which were drawn on and amplified as the case progressed. I then track three distinct but overlapping early constructions of Fisher's character that are relevant to understanding his initial fall from grace before considering the tragic-hero-turned-vindicated-visionary persona, which melds together key elements of his earlier representations. I conclude the chapter by considering what characterizations of Fisher suggest about the ethos of science in an age of large-scale federal funding and oversight. But first, to understand how constructions of Fisher's character affected the contours of the controversy, we must visit Pittsburgh in the decades before the first glimmers of controversy arose, when Fisher was transitioning from his boyhood in the city's Squirrel Hill neighborhood to his scientific career on its flagship campus.

THE MAKING OF A (PITTSBURGH) SCIENTIST

Although much of the early newspaper coverage painted portraits of a "fallen" hero, an "embattled" doctor, or a career gone awry, a sympathetic portrayal of Fisher appeared in the *Pittsburgh Post-Gazette* nine months after Datagate boiled over.[7] Because the account offered details of Fisher's life leading up to his work for NSABP, I use it as a launching point to discuss his career and to stress his long-term connection to the University of Pittsburgh, interspersing it with other biographical sources. The idea is to show how his early efforts crafted a revolutionary scientific persona that played into dominant media frames. For example, the *Post-Gazette* account romanticized the story of a young man attracted to science from his earliest years when he would stay home from school reading books such as Paul de Kruif's *Microbe Hunters* when, less romantically, he faced frequent bouts of whooping cough, scarlet fever, measles, and mumps.[8] The *Post-Gazette* conveyed a sense of the significance of science in Fisher's formative years acknowledging key influences in Fisher's life, including his great-uncle Julius Rogoff, a well-known Case Western University surgeon and physiologist, and high school chemistry teacher Lon Colburn. It offered a tale of the American dream, as Fisher and his brother, Edwin, the progeny of Lithuanian immigrants who ran a produce shop, grew up in the shadow of the University of Pittsburgh's Cathedral of Learning and eventually rose to its towering heights.

Anticipating the drama of the eventual forced separation from his longtime academic home, the *Post-Gazette* stressed Fisher's decades-long affiliation with the university, which began when, as a young boy in the 1920s, he contributed ten cents to the building of the Cathedral of Learning, the university's forty-five-story Gothic skyscraper that came to dominate the landscape in Oakland, Pittsburgh's then-fledgling cultural and educational center. The mention of Fisher's connection to the university, his childhood donation to the Cathedral of Learning, rendered a pathos-laden scene, suggesting how ignominious his separation from Pittsburgh must have been. Indeed, Fisher spent most of his academic career at the university, earning his baccalaureate in 1936, a chemistry degree in 1939, and a medical degree in 1943, and he retains his connection to Pitt this day.[9] When an ulcer prevented him from serving in World War II, he interned at nearby Mercy Hospital, soon marrying Shirley Krum, a bacteriologist who then worked at Pittsburgh's West Penn Hospital. Fisher continued postgraduate training in Pittsburgh before stints at the University of Pennsylvania and Hammersmith Hospital in London. He did not stay away from his alma mater for long, however, and returned in 1952 as a Markle Scholar in Medical Science, an honor that recognized his exceptional promise.[10] In short, the boy who had grown up in Squirrel Hill was assembling the elements of future scientific stardom. By 1958, a mere thirteen years out of medical school, he had contributed to nearly fifty academic publications while working in two laboratories at Pitt. The first was in an attic of the old Mellon Institute on O'Hara Street in Oakland, where Fisher had established a laboratory for experimental surgery. The second was located in room 914, Scaife Hall, in the building where he would work for the bulk of his career and where he would return for his Legacy Laureate lecture. His annual operating budget for research when he started was roughly fifty thousand dollars, but his interest in breast cancer research would come later.[11]

Although Fisher had published an essay called "Supraradical Cancer Surgery," in the *American Journal of Surgery* in 1954, he has explicitly stated that when his career began, he "had no interest in chemotherapy, clinical trials, or breast cancer."[12] According to the standard story, when chief surgeon Dr. George Moore of Roswell Park in Buffalo telephoned Fisher in 1955 and asked him to join the cancer institute he was founding, Fisher claims to have declined, saying, "I am not really interested in cancer."[13] Yet, three years later, in 1958, Fisher's mentor Isidor S. Ravdin reportedly called from the University of Pennsylvania and said, "We're having a meeting in Washington at the National Institutes of Health, and I want you to be there." Ravdin explained, "We're going to set up a clinical trial involving women with breast cancer."[14] Fisher recalled his reply was something along the lines of, "I'm not in the least bit interested. I'm doing what I want to do in the laboratory here at Pitt."[15] When Ravdin responded, "I'm telling you to be there," Fisher acquiesced. As he later explained in an interview with Leah Kauffman of *Pitt Med Magazine*, "You don't refuse a two-star general who . . . had operated on

Eisenhower, and who was known the world over."[16] Elsewhere, he has joked, "*No one* refused his orders."[17]

The meeting, which took place in Stone House (Building 16) on the NIH campus, would "profoundly change" Fisher's professional life, even though he claims to have gone "reluctantly."[18] "I considered the endeavor a distraction that would interfere with my studies on liver regeneration,'" he explained.[19] The meeting at Stone House concerned NIH-sponsored research that sought to investigate anecdotal evidence from the 1950s that chemotherapy following surgery could improve cancer patient outcomes. The research was to be conducted as part of the "Surgical Adjuvant Chemotherapy Projects" under the auspices of the NIH's Cancer Chemotherapy National Service Center (CCNSC).[20] Fisher noted, "It was there that I became aware of the paucity of investigation into how cancer cells disseminated" and that Ravdin proposed a clunky title, the National Surgical Adjuvant Breast and Bowel Project, for what the group was proposing to do: conduct the first-ever breast adjuvant chemotherapy trial.[21] Despite his later becoming a self-labeled "clinical trials zealot," the proposed research interested Fisher only slightly. He told the *Pittsburgh Post-Gazette* in 1994, "I said, 'Oh, what the hell, OK.'"[22] However, for a man who professed not to have had any initial interest in cancer or clinical trials, Fisher soon became a convert. "I became wedded to the clinical trial concept," he recounted.[23] That same year, the first clinical trial began under the NSABP banner, enrolling 826 patients within the first three years.[24] Fisher would later describe these early years as "halcyon days when money was plentiful and the freedom to pursue one's own research interests was unbridled."[25] Such freedom and excitement provided the opportunity for Fisher to carve out a place for himself in a new current of biomedical thinking.

When Bernard Fisher became chair of the NSABP in the late 1950s, the idea of using clinical trials to prove the efficacy of surgeries for breast cancer was new. Fisher had to persuade his colleagues that clinical trials were necessary to determine the success of surgical options for breast cancer, and his audience was recalcitrant. But first Fisher himself had to seize on the idea, for breast cancer surgery at the time was generally not regarded a proper subject for clinical trial experimentation. Surgeons expressed the view that removing women's breasts was tantamount to necessary battery. Some felt that surgical removal of the breasts and pectoral muscles was harmful enough, and that experimenting on women with surgical procedures whose efficacy was unknown probably constituted a violation of medical ethics. Although surgical innovations have long been the subject of professional disputation, Fisher argued that they needed to undergo the rigors of testing. In so doing, he took on the surgical establishment in a way that built his reputation and secured his place in oncological history, but also created a persona of a revolutionary, albeit one whose voice was inflected with brash arrogance. Regardless of whether he knew at the time that he was forging the persona of revolutionary, Fisher increasingly cultivated this persona in later life as he drew explicitly on Thomas Kuhn's rhetoric of paradigm shifts to describe his role in changing breast cancer treatment science.[26] But first the old paradigm had to show cracks. In order for Fisher to persuade others of the value of the rigors of clinical research, the seeds for this change had to be firmly planted in the biomedical imagination.

THE FOUR FACES OF BERNARD FISHER

Fisher as Swashbuckling Scientific Revolutionary: Dissident Surgeon or Hero?

Decades before he was called to testify before Congress concerning his management of NSABP, Bernard Fisher mounted a challenge against surgical orthodoxy. More specifically, he questioned the theory that breast cancer spreads outward from the tumor site. But perhaps more heretically, his challenge threatened to dislodge the regnant Halsted radical mastectomy, one of the most enduring and deeply entrenched surgeries in the history of U.S. medicine. As a result, intense battles between Fisher and the surgical establishment ensued. As medical historian Barron Lerner would later assert, Fisher became the "bane of breast surgeons."[27] The predominant media frame during the initial days of Datagate drew from Fisher's reputed stormy relation to the old-guard surgical orthodoxy to position him as a revolutionary whose renegade actions made him ripe for a downfall. Thus, as we shall soon discover, Fisher's performance of the scientific revolutionary was accomplished with a swagger. Early efforts of self-construction as a paradigm-busting revolutionary catapulted Fisher to fame, to be sure, but they also left him exposed to the attacks of those with old scores to settle. Fisher created this persona, albeit perhaps unwittingly, when he mounted an attack on the dominant surgical treatment for breast cancer of the twentieth century, the surgically favored but painful and disfiguring Halsted method.

Even as the Halsted mastectomy became deeply entrenched as the standard of care for breast cancer in the middle of the twentieth century, a story we read in chapter 1, lingering doubts led some surgeons to question its ubiquitous use. This aspect is important to understand because Fisher's actions within the context of challenges to the dominant Halsted surgery primed colleagues to view him with a mixture of awe and disdain. For some he was a hero, an icon to be emulated and admired, while others regarded him with extreme derision. Lerner's account of how Fisher's early years positioned him antagonistically to the surgical orthodoxy, which overwhelmingly favored Halsted, is instructive. Lerner recounted that on October 14, 1970, debates about the Halsted approach pervaded the fifty-sixth annual congress of the American College of Surgeons in Chicago. One brave surgeon, George "Barney" Crile, presented retrospective data suggesting that simple mastectomies and lumpectomies produced survival rates as high as the Halsted radical mastectomy. Crile observed that European surgeons were abandoning Halsted, and he argued that the time had come for women to have a say in what kind of treatment they should have. Lerner explained that "audience reaction was as vociferous as ever. 'Are you kidding?' asked the first questioner, to peals of laughter."[28] A second questioner asked, "Does any reputable surgical figure in this country besides Dr. Crile support the concept of a limited mastectomy and irradiation?"[29] While Crile "won points for his courage and candor," the "star of the show," in Lerner's account, was Bernard Fisher.[30] After years of unsuccessfully trying to convince surgeons to study their methods scientifically, Fisher finally made headway in Chicago. Instead of their usual derision, the audience applauded Fisher's closing statement: "I believe that all of us must get these clinical trials done as quickly as possible and not sit on our butts and continue year after year to go through this same type of masturbation."[31]

Accusing his colleagues of laziness and pointless self-stimulation was sure to draw both ire and admiring smirks. The rhetorical tone, the voice, of Fisher's self-presentation in the years leading up to his success is significant. Although many of his exact words have floated away in the manner of all oral presentations, Lerner recounted that "Fisher had the stereotypical personality of a surgeon."[32] He was "confrontational and self assured often to the point of arrogance."[33] At meetings, he stood and "importuned" in a "sonorous and authoritative voice."[34] On top of that, the choices he made in presenting the content of his message were sure to ruffle feathers. He railed against the "miasma of mediocrity" that pervaded clinical oncology.[35] In his calls for a more limited surgery, he "was thoroughly upsetting the applecart."[36] In short, "Bernie" Fisher was brazen, bold, and highly heretical. Further compounding matters, Fisher existed in a liminal zone. Unlike Crile, who was himself a surgeon, Fisher was partly a surgeon, partly a researcher; this hybrid role further separated him from many more mainstream, conventional surgeons. Recognizing the distance between them, he once remarked that surgeons did not quite know what to make of him.[37]

Thus, Fisher carved out a new role, the "surgical oncologist," and spent years convincing others to join him.

The brash persona Fisher had forged early in his career and the threat he posed to the surgical orthodoxy were met by attempts by others to thwart his efforts. Fisher had a very difficult time recruiting patients for his clinical trials in the 1970s, partially because he had alienated influential surgeons like Cushman Haagenson, who had warned that physicians risked "ruination of the soul" if they followed Fisher, whom Haagenson dubbed "a dissident surgeon."[38] Journalist Mackenzie Carpenter drew on this backstory during Datagate to inform readers that "beating up on Fisher—at least verbally—was a popular sport for members of the American surgical establishment in the 1950s and 60s."[39] This strained relationship with members of the surgical old guard meant that Fisher spent years trying to recruit enough patients for his lumpectomy trials, taking to the road to find smaller clinics, since the larger ones would not endorse his project. He ended up recruiting at places like Johnstown and Oil City, Pennsylvania, and Wichita Falls, Texas. Finally, in 1971 he had enough patients to begin a trial of comparative surgery, NSABP's Project B-04, which measured outcomes of radical mastectomy against simple mastectomy, which left the pectoral walls in place. When Fisher presented his results at a National Cancer Institute conference in 1974, he was "flushed with success." However, he would later note that that feeling lasted for only twenty-four hours, because colleagues "trashed him."[40] When low enrollment rates in his early trials, such as Datagate's influential lumpectomy trial, led him to develop prerandomization as a way of upping his enrollment numbers, statisticians lambasted his scientific rigor.[41]

Over the years, Fisher repeatedly demarcated his brand of breast cancer research from the orthodoxy by stressing the "science" of randomized clinical trials as superior to the anecdotal happenstance of days past, a move that solidified his status as a vanguard of change. Fisher insisted that the "anecdotal" explanations of Halsted supporters "had little enduring impact because they contained no special concept or scientific principle that could be subject to further testing and future investigation."[42] In 1993 he explained that "Physicians currently influenced by the Halstedian paradigm are being governed by the science of a previous era." Despite Halsted's innovations, Fisher insisted that insights derived from Halsted's accounts "were each nothing more than a cul-de-sac!"[43] With a voice of superiority, he thus drew a sharp contrast between the well-grounded practices of a man of science and the hunches of the anecdotalist. Rhetoricians Kenneth Zagacki and William Keith have noted that labeling oneself as "scientific" in contrast to one's "non-scientific" predecessors is a stock topos of the revolutionary persona.[44] And indeed, Fisher pitted his scientific approach against that of many of his colleagues. Both his 1985 *World Journal of Surgery* article "The Revolution in Breast Cancer Surgery: Science or Anecdotalism?" and his 1991 essay "The Importance of Clinical Trials," cast the anecdotal approach as unworthy for the new science of clinical trials. "By replacing anecdotal information (which has influenced therapeutic decision making in the past) with more credible and substantive data," he argued, "clinical trials play a major role in transforming the practice of medicine from an art to a science."[45] Whereas many of his colleagues were "merely" offering retrospective analysis, Fisher was engaged in the more noble pursuit of laboratory studies. "During the time that the anecdotal clinical information was accumulating," he observed, "we were carrying out a series of laboratory and clinical investigations."[46] By contrast to the others, "our efforts were directed toward obtaining a better comprehension of the biology of metastases."[47] Fisher positioned his endeavor as better than that of his anecdotalist peers, labeling their retrospective trials "worthless," "unsystematic," and "non-science."[48] Fisher thus cast himself as a scientist par excellence, a bulwark against a tide of amateurism and anecdotalism.

Fisher's rhetoric increasingly adopted a Kuhnian stance of "revolutions" and "paradigm shifts" when he described the move from Halstedian tenets to the alternative hypothesis that he, among others, posited. These statements referred, of course, to Thomas Kuhn's *Structure of Scientific Revolutions,* which contrasted "normal science," in which the existence of a paradigm would determine the kind of questions that are examined in science, with a "scientific revolution," which would challenge an existing paradigm and force the emergence of a new one. As early as 1985, for example, he wrote that "During the past 15 to 20 years, there have resulted revolutionary changes in the local/regional management of primary breast cancer."[49] Echoing this theme, two years before the Datagate controversy reverberated through the mass media Fisher penned a *Cancer Research* essay, "The Evolution of Paradigms for the Management of Breast Cancer: A Personal Perspective," in which he explicitly enrolled Kuhn's notion of paradigms to explain his and NSABP's contributions to cancer research.[50] One year later, in 1993, he similarly argued that "during the past two decades a revolution has occurred in the surgical treatment of primary breast cancer." By presenting his alternative hypothesis—"The Fisher Hypothesis," as it came to be known—as a radical rupture rather than a gradual change, he was symbolically able to cement his position in a scientific sea change. When discussing the "paradigm" that gave rise to Halsted, he explained that "a second, alternative hypothesis, which I synthesized almost 25 years ago contends that cancer is a systemic disease." In another essay, he wrote, "In 1970 after an extensive evaluation of the reports, I concluded that the material presented had not demonstrated that the extended radical procedure was more efficacious than the conventional radical mastectomy."[51] Fisher's rhetoric thus obscured a competing discourse of gradualism wherein the Halsted method was dislodged by women's refusal to consent to breast removal, and by scores of physicians and dozens of published studies that argued for systemic theories of cancer. In Fisher's revolutionary frame, these factors could be explained as a response to his paradigm-busting vision rather than as key contributors to the coming change. Although Fisher presented his ideas as decidedly revolutionary, other possible accounts could easily have stressed a more gradual, more widely collaborative, and nonrevolutionary effort.

Fisher's calls for a "rational basis" for breast cancer treatment, as we have seen, form part of a recurrent theme invoked over several decades. This strategy proved effective on three levels. First, it established a new standard of proof—randomized clinical trials—and not the existing "proof" of retrospective analyses and anecdotal evidence. Second, it positioned Fisher as someone who could supply the needed proof, thus securing his position in the history of breast cancer research. Third, it allowed him to assume the persona of a pathbreaking scientist, a revolutionary, who significantly altered the course of scientific progress. As it turned out, that persona came into being through antagonism to the surgical orthodoxy, which as Zagacki and Keith have noted, could potentially occur through the use of revolutionary, conciliatory, or conservative stances.[52] One of the undercurrents of Fisher's construction of himself as carrier of the scientific mantle, and of the surgical orthodoxy's opposition to his efforts, was that Fisher's calls for a more limited surgery threatened to challenge surgical authority. That surgeons recognized and attempted to contain this perceived threat is evident in their belittling Fisher's surgical prowess, lobbing criticisms that he "could not operate his way out of a paper bag."[53] As Datagate unfolded, Fisher would draw from these early clashes to claim persecution by the surgical establishment, a characterization that endured in his rhetoric. In the Legacy Laureate speech discussed in the opening of this chapter, which Fisher delivered in 2000, the scientist implicitly compared his experience to the persecution of Galileo—a not so humble comparison that resonated with previous constructions of hubris.[54]

Six years earlier, as news of Datagate spread, widely circulating accounts drew from his past reputation to cast Fisher as a scientific revolutionary of the swashbuckling variety. On April 4, 1994, the *New York Times* article "Fall of a Man Pivotal in Breast Cancer Research," by science writer Lawrence K. Altman, affirmed Fisher's great stature while simultaneously stressing his arrogance. It portrayed Fisher as following "his own agenda," and noted that he "might not have accepted every piece of advice that was offered to him," observing his "refusal to take advice or heed instructions from his bureaucratic masters." The article noted that Fisher bore himself in a "manner that is often perceived as arrogant and abrasive." The *Times* used the terms *strong* or *forceful* nine times when describing Fisher's personality.[55] By contrast, the *Pittsburgh Post-Gazette's* local coverage by Steve Twedt was a bit more circumspect, even as it echoed a portrait of swashbuckling arrogance. The *Pittsburgh Post-Gazette's* "3 Weeks Shake Cancer Pioneer's 30-Year Record" emphasized Fisher's eminence and "pioneering" status, with the words *pioneer* or *pioneering* occurring more than four times along with labels such as "giant" and "hero." Fisher was cast as a "straight shooter" who possessed "intellectual integrity." And yet, he was "arrogant," "abrupt," "disdainful of non-scientists," and "abrupt with those who take opposing views to his," a characterization that reinforced his arrogance. That Fisher made important strides in breast cancer research is clear, but when juxtaposed with descriptions such as "abrasive," "abrupt," and "not to be pushed around," the article sustained a verbal portrait of arrogance.[56] Fisher is not only responsible for prompting major changes in science, for being a revolutionary, he is a swashbuckling revolutionary, an arrogant revolutionary, and these perceived traits haunted efforts to restore his reputation by providing inventional fodder to his critics and by undercutting trust in his management skills and by extension his scientific findings. Table 1 outlines the major clusters of character references in these two articles, which is instructive about how past perceptions of his character, honed during his days fighting the surgical establishment, reappeared during Datagate.

Strains of the revolutionary persona previously forged by Fisher appeared in these articles in terms of his "pioneer" status, his role in changing breast cancer research, and his "giant" or "heroic" stature. Fisher, in short, was symbolically cast as a scientific icon credited with "single-handedly" changing dominant views of cancer, with "fundament(ally) reshaping breast cancer treatment." The revolutionary persona reinforced what rhetorician Davida Charney has called the "myth of the lone genius," the idea that one man—and it usually is assumed to be a man—alone changes science.[57] Characterizations of Fisher here emphasized his strength, arrogance, forcefulness, and unwillingness to listen to or cooperate with others. The vision of science encapsulated in the revolutionary persona is predicated on contest and overthrow rather than cooperation and communalism. In the case of Datagate, critics marshaled Fisher's personality traits of strength and self-assurance to maintain that he was unfit to manage the NSABP, even as his defenders pitched the same traits as evidence of his devotion to his science. Nonetheless, it is important to note that it was not the revolutionary persona alone

Table 1. Verbal Portraits of a Man: A Comparison of Fisher's Character in Two Newspaper Articles from April 1994

Source and Author	*New York Times* "Fall of a Man Pivotal in Breast Cancer Research" by Lawrence K. Altman	*Pittsburgh Post-Gazette* "3 Weeks Shake Cancer Pioneer's 30-Year Record" by Steve Twedt
Descriptive Clusters		
Changed Breast Cancer Treatment/ Research	Pivotal (*headline*) pivotal "single-handedly has done more to change our perception of breast cancer than any other single individual in the world"	fundamentally reshaped (breast cancer treatment) "man who has done so much in the field of breast cancer research" "won just about every major scientific prize short of the Nobel" accomplish(ments) "Mr. Breast Cancer" (said "in tones of deep respect")
Giant/Hero		Giant Hero heroic "almost a hero in the 1970s" "Dr. Fisher also believes he's a hero"
Pioneer	"pioneering large-scale research"	Cancer Pioneer (*headline*) pioneer pioneering pioneer(ing work) has done "more than any other researcher" to fight for breast cancer

Source and Author	*New York Times* "Fall of a Man Pivotal in Breast Cancer Research" by Lawrence K. Altman	*Pittsburgh Post-Gazette* "3 Weeks Shake Cancer Pioneer's 30-Year Record" by Steve Twedt
Descriptive Clusters		
Strong/Forceful/ Arrogant	'A Strong Personality' (*section heading*)	"a tough guy to deal with"
	strong personality (*twice*)	arrogant
	driving person	
	strong personality	
	strong in his views	
	forceful (personality)	
	forceful(ness of being right)	
	"self-confident with a manner that is often perceived as arrogant and abrasive"	
	outspoken, very clear, strong in his views	
	"clearly not to be pushed around" (by the vicissitudes of smaller issues)	
Insular/Self-Driven	"had his own agenda"	disdainful of non-scientists
	"might not have accepted every piece of advice that was offered to him"	"abrupt with those who take views opposing his"
	"refusal to take advice or heed instructions from his bureaucratic masters"	"(I think) he thinks some of these things like breast cancer support groups are extraneous"
		"he doesn't have much patience (with breast cancer support groups)"

Continued on the next page

Table 1. *Continued*

Source and Author	*New York Times* "Fall of a Man Pivotal in Breast Cancer Research" by Lawrence K. Altman	*Pittsburgh Post-Gazette* "3 Weeks Shake Cancer Pioneer's 30-Year Record" by Steve Twedt
Descriptive Clusters		
Insular/Self-Driven (*continued*)		"and doesn't think he needs to listen to anyone else"
		"likes to keep it in the scientific arena, not the political arena"
Effective Leader/ Organizer	"knows how to discipline others"	"dynamic in terms of leadership"
	"able to effectively run meetings with hundreds of people and to plan programs"	
	"success in providing hard answers to vexing questions"	
	organizer of vast clinical trials	
Honest (Intellectually)	"(had a) great deal of character"	"straightest shooter to ever walk a hospital corridor"
		intellectual integrity
		intellectual honesty
		"interest(ed) in pursuing things above board"

that provided material for attacks on or defenses of Fisher, but the amplified, albeit perhaps distorted, echoes of his formerly brash and swaggering voice that became the basis for concern. As one writer put it, "Dr. Fisher's own arrogance has contributed to his downfall. He acted as though he had no obligation to the women who participate in his trials and to the public which provides the funding."[58]

Indeed, perceptions of Fisher's arrogance spilled over into other contexts, hampering his attempts to clear his name. When called to testify before Congress and interviewed in various outlets, federal and local officials referred to Fisher's arrogance as evidence that he was responsible for bad oversight. Thus, his character trait is linked to his integrity as a knowledge producer. Some officials used the trope of "formidable patriarch" to explain why no one had initially questioned him concerning his management of NSABP. For instance, the *Lancet* explained that "NCI's civil servants ... were intimidated by Fisher the patriarch of enlightened breast-cancer treatment, possessor of a 'formidable intellect' and of 'formidable renown.'" NCI's Sam Broder stated, "sorrowfully" in science reporter Daniel Greenberg's estimation, that Fisher's response to the NCI "was quite disrespectful of the role that government employees play and quite disrespectful of the status and functions that we have."[59] Broder recounted that Fisher "'said words to the effect of who are you to criticize me. I know how to do clinical trials. I've been doing them before you were a doctor.'"[60] This statement, made in response to an NCI request for new auditing procedures in 1992, solidified a picture of Fisher as someone who thought he was not accountable to others in the scientific community.

Pittsburgh officials cited a "culture of deference" that prevented them from questioning Fisher or demanding more oversight. This construction is linked to Fisher's perceived revolutionary status, which overseers used as an explanation for why they did not question his capacity to lead the NSABP. Toward the end of the congressional testimony of Dr. Thomas Detre, senior vice chancellor of health sciences at the University of Pittsburgh, at the first of two Dingell hearings, Congressman Sherrod Brown reintroduced the "culture of deference" theme mentioned in Detre's testimony:

Mr. Brown: Dr. Detre, in your prepared statement, you spoke about the culture of deference.

Mr. Detre: Yes, sir.

Mr. Brown: Culture of deference in academic settings toward a university senior scientist, something that obviously—I would think—is not unique to the University of Pittsburgh certainly. Did that culture of deference at Pittsburgh toward Dr. Fisher, did that contribute to the university's failure of oversight?

Mr. Detre: I believe it contributes to any university's failure because we don't have any mechanism in place to truly supervise senior faculty. Our expectation, Congressman Brown, is that if there are problems, they will be reported by the senior faculty member to

the chairman of the department and, through him, to the dean; but
clearly, this mechanism alone is insufficient.

Mr. Brown: You told the subcommittee staff in an informal survey
that 90 percent of Pittsburgh's academic peers treat senior scientists in a sort of similar hands-off, detached fashion in a sense. Is
this, in fact, a problem throughout the university?[61]

Although Detre attempted to sidestep the issue in his answers to this
line of questioning, his response implied that University of Pittsburgh officials were reluctant to challenge Fisher because of his perceived status at
the pinnacle of the medical pantheon. This move invoked existing constructions of Fisher as the brash, untouchable revolutionary. After years of fighting to achieve recognition and acceptance, Fisher's pathbreaking position
would ultimately be used against him. He had become a towering edifice of
science, but his success rested on a perceived foundation of arrogance and
thus made him a suitable target for scapegoating, particularly among those
who remembered his early days. As Craig Henderson of the University of
California at San Francisco opined, members of the surgical old guard "were
raised to think of Bernard Fisher as the bogeyman, and these things take a
long time to die."[62]

Thus, the dominant construction of Fisher to unfold in the early weeks
of Datagate inflected the revolutionary persona with more than a tinge of
bravura, thereby consolidating the perception that Fisher was arrogant and
fueling criticisms that he withheld critical information from American
women. The revolutionary persona therefore embedded the ethos of science in an individualized context. It registered not only the collective ro-
mance with the myth of the lone genius, toiling away in solitary pursuit of
big ideals, but also public frustration with those who seem to disregard their
interests and needs. This persona thus undermined public trust in NSABP
research, and by synecdochic extension, all federally funded research. However, while the swashbuckling revolutionary served as a dominant recircu-
lation of existing accounts of Fisher's character, this persona was in contest
with another construction that shattered the revolutionary mythos and exposed the underbelly of big science.

Fisher as Beleaguered Bureaucrat

The second major persona that vied for legitimacy during Datagate featured
Fisher the beleaguered bureaucrat of science. To be sure, Fisher faced formidable administrative pressures that would have inevitably accompanied
the now sprawling NSABP. These duties would have only increased further

after news of Poisson's falsifications. It is therefore not surprising that Fisher himself first raised the issue of multiplying administrative duties as a reason for his slowness in publishing a reanalysis of the data from B-06 or his continuing to submit essays with Poisson data, one of the more serious charges leveled against him. Fisher planted seeds for the beleaguered bureaucrat characterization when he observed that the preceding years had become particularly hectic. His April 13, 1994, statement to the House Oversight Committee noted that "the number of patients being followed in NSABP studies" had "increased from 25,000 in 1991 to 41,000 in 1993."[63] Moreover, he testified to a data explosion, explaining that "the number of data forms processed expanded from 225,000 in 1991 to 413,000 in 1993."[64] NSABP's thirty-five years coincided with the burgeoning of clinical biomedical research wherein increased professionalization of medicine pushed bureaucracy, the rise of clinical trials entailed more paperwork and regulations, and the growing demand for patient participation in trials meant higher enrollment and management demands. In light of the complexity and scope of the NSABP, its large number of investigators, its rapid expansion, and its complex relationships to multiple governing agencies, it is little wonder that the persona of beleaguered bureaucrat surfaced. Although Fisher himself initially offered administrative duties as a reason for his delay in publishing reanalyses of Poisson's data, Dingell and other critics wielded his delay as evidence that Fisher was overwhelmed by his group's day-to-day operations. Amplified in media accounts, this persona made Fisher appear negligent at the same time that it exposed the fact that the biomedical community lacked precedent for how to respond to the complexities of the situation before them, and that the demands of a highly bureaucratized science called for new ways of thinking and acting.

In many ways, Fisher's stature and the nature of allegations against him made him a desirable target of John Dingell's zealous pursuit of big science in the mid-1990s. Fisher's appearance at Dingell's oversight hearing provided support for the view that Fisher was not in command of the daily operations of his organization. At one point, Dingell began questioning Fisher about NSABP audit reports. "Of course, Doctor," Dingell observed, "these went to eligibility and showed there were some fairly significant eligibility questions. For example, one site had three-quarters of the participants ineligible."[65] Fisher's response was heartbreaking:

> Mr. Fisher: I am certainly unaware of that, sir. I really am not aware
>   of it.
> Mr. Dingell: But it was in audit reports that came to you, though.
> Mr. Fisher: I don't, I really don't remember seeing that report at all.

Mr. Dingell: Well, here they are, and I am just going to lay them out. South Nassau Hospital, Rush Presbyterian Hospital, St. Joseph in Lancaster, and in the University of Pittsburgh. Now, the University of California Davis had ¾ of the participants in the study ineligible.

Mr. Fisher: I have never seen these.

Mr. Dingell: These were audits, these were audits in your project.

[The discussion continued with Fisher discussing the nature of clinical trial eligibility requirements.]

Mr. Fisher: I certainly am not aware of any institution where there were ¾ of the patients ineligible. I should like to have more information about that than I have.

Mr. Dingell: Well, we will give it to you. It is, however, I would observe, Doctor, in your own audit reports. Now, here are other examples. Auditors turned up instances where patients were randomized twice. What is the result of randomizing a patient twice in a study of this kind? What does it do to the statistical validity of the study?

Mr. Fisher: I can't answer that question.

[Dingell continued to question Fisher about a number of matters.]

Mr. Fisher: Sir, I cannot answer these questions unless I know the specific cases and so on. I am sorry. We continue to try to educate these people.

Mr. Dingell: It is my impression that you were the man that ran this whole thing.[66]

This blistering lashing, this seemingly damning evidence, must have felt devastating to Fisher. Here appeared to be a man unaware of the content of his own outfit's audits! Here appeared to be a man who could not answer questions about eligibility requirements of the trials he had run! And most disturbing of all, here appeared to be a scientist who seemingly could not address the statistical validity of his eligibility requirements! Yet this interchange between two powerful men reveals the tensions between big science, wherein scientific giants are reduced to paper pushers facing an endless parade of reports, and politics, where accountability and transparency become token topoi wielded over others during times of crisis. On the one hand, for critics, this line of inquiry made Fisher appear blindingly incompetent—for he could not even address the perils of double randomization. But on the other hand, Dingell's expectation that Fisher would know the details of numerous audits during a time of great duress—after enduring near-daily beatings in the media, the loss of his beloved position at NSABP, and the countless other indignities he faced—defies the limits of human endurance. Nonetheless, when viewed from a public sphere frame, as opposed to a technical frame, Fisher's inability to appear in command of his organization conveyed the persona of a beleaguered bureaucrat drowning in a sea of case reports and methodological minutiae. Rather than adopting a voice of contrition or supplication, he appeared, on the one hand, defiant and yet, on the other, defeated, out of touch, and besieged. "It was clear," said Michael Friedman, who directed the NCI's cancer therapy evaluation program, "that Dr. Fisher was being overwhelmed by the workload."[67] Yet, for his supporters, it was also clear that Fisher was unfairly paraded around Washington in a skirmish over science that was larger than the NSABP.

Amplifying broader themes of big science run amok, unchecked and extravagant, the *Washington Post* report "Researcher Accused of 'Lavish Parties'" replayed another damaging line of questioning from the Dingell hearing:

> "It does appear to me that you are more expansive with your expenditures for parties than you are for auditing," Dingell told Fisher at one point near the end of nearly two hours at the witness table.
>
> Fisher seemed to shrink in his seat, shrugged and said, "After a lifetime of dedication to science, I find that absolutely devastating."[68]

Fisher's appearance—his slumping, shrugging, and seeming inability to answer questions—accentuated the beleaguered bureaucrat persona, reinforcing the view that he was overwhelmed by volumes of paperwork and out of touch with the needs of breast cancer patients. It fostered a powerful perception of mismanagement for his critics at the same time that it reinforced perceptions of the unfairness of the mediated political spectacle to Fisher's supporters.

Whereas at the second hearing Fisher bravely attempted to answer Dingell's questions, he had sent a written statement to the April 13, 1994, session in lieu of appearing in person (a decision with devastating consequences that will be considered in the next subsection of this chapter). Although his statement was omitted from the published hearing transcripts, it was reprinted in the April 22, 1994, *Cancer Letter*. "Having directed the National Surgical Adjuvant Breast & Bowel Project for over 25 years," Fisher began, "I am now engaged in a comprehensive evaluation of the issues raised by recent disclosures."[69] Here, Fisher attempted to convey his command of NSABP operations, to take responsibility for determining what went wrong. Fisher stressed the significance of NSABP breast cancer research by explicitly appealing to the revolutionary nature of NSABP findings. "The findings from our trials," he explained, "have revolutionized the treatment of this dread disease by demonstrating that lumpectomy followed by radiation therapy, rather than a disfiguring radical mastectomy, is the preferable treatment for most women with breast cancer."[70] Seeking to further his and NSABP's credibility, Fisher reviewed influential NSABP research findings before matter-of-factly recounting his 1991 discovery: "We found that an investigator from St. Luc Hospital in Montreal had deliberately altered data relating to patient eligibility for clinical trials."[71] Moreover, "we immediately informed the NCI," and "promptly reanalyzed the studies in which patients from St. Luc hospital had participated."[72]

Despite his efforts to cast himself as having acted quickly and properly, amid charges that he continued to submit data from Poisson that he knew was tainted, Fisher faced a mountain of criticism that an earnest recounting of his actions alone could scarcely counter. Moreover, his rationale for his delay in publishing a reanalysis of the B-06 data without Poisson's numbers provided the basis for a later sedimentation of the persona of the beleaguered bureaucrat. Fisher explained that he had not published a reanalysis of Poisson's data, because he believed other NSABP projects to be of higher priority and because auditing procedures were underfunded. Moreover, he noted that his workload had multiplied since the initiation of the much-celebrated breast cancer prevention trial: "In the past 18 months, our work has expanded enormously. A newly initiated breast cancer prevention trial recruited more patients in one year than were recruited in any year in all of the treatment trials combined."[73] With now more than five hundred sites participating in NSABP data collection, processing, and analysis, the success of the NSABP—its size, its scope, and its influence—and its consolidation under one strong leader would also be its weakness. How could any one person ensure that hundreds of data collection sites with varying personnel were all conforming to the rules? At various times during the controversy, Fisher further stressed that he had not been allowed to talk about the case.[74]

The persona of the beleaguered bureaucrat/scientific administrator rests on a role tension that could either evoke sympathy for Fisher's deluge of work or bolster the view that he was derelict in his duties because he misjudged the seriousness of the threat to the credibility of the data. Amid newspaper reports that "Fisher . . . said he had fallen into a deep depression after being forced to step down in late March as head of the project," Fisher sympathizers might have felt that their man was unfairly being asked to account for too much.[75] Fisher told the press that "'after being and doing what I did for so many years, and then suddenly one day [to be] called and told I was no longer going to be chairman of this thing, and there was no due process or anything else, that was a devastating thing for me.'"[76] Although these statements offered insight into the mounting pressures Fisher faced, they are consistent with the perception that he was overwhelmed and reinforced the idea that the situation at the NSABP was not properly managed.

Newspapers pushed this perception to broader audiences. The *New York Times* featured a story about Fisher that emphasized his administrative backlog less than a week after his failure to appear at the first Dingell hearing. Especially resonant was the voice of NCI's Dr. Bruce A. Chabner, who noted that Fisher had "failed to respond to 'five or six' written requests to publish his reanalysis of the lumpectomy study without the Poisson data." "Dr. Fisher's team was a year behind in visits to cooperating hospitals to audit their data and was extremely slow to report to the cancer institute serious deficiencies found in the audits," Chabner continued. Moreover, "The fact that they were so far behind was not tolerable," and "Bernie just was not responding."[77] These statements reveal how the persona of the reluctant apologist, to which we will turn in the next section of the chapter, dovetailed with that of the beleaguered bureaucrat to create a picture of an overwhelmed, negligent scientist who was unable to oversee a burgeoning organization. The credibility contest now hinged on which persona, and which accompanying narrative of responsibility, with its attendant moral judgments, would reign. And another potentially damning construction of Fisher offered a slightly different, albeit equally vexing, frame.

Fisher as Reluctant Apologist in Two Senses

A third characterization presented the face of a reluctant apologist. This persona resulted from the interplay of Fisher's own voice with that of other scientists and administrators. Fisher himself enacted the role of reluctant apologist in two senses. In one sense, his silence during crucial moments of the controversy did not satisfy public or congressional demands for contrition. His seeming refusal to apologize for his failure to notify publics when he first learned of Poisson's faulty data or to stop publishing B-06 results struck some as unforgiveable, even if some members of the scientific community defended this stance as scientifically defensible.[78] In a stronger sense, Fisher refused to apologize for the vagaries of big science or for science's putative separation from public life. To be fair, part of his perceived reluctance to apologize can be understood as a response to the truculent, turbulent political climate that participants in big science found themselves in the mid-1990s: Fisher was hardly the first big-name scientist called to testify before Dingell's subcommittee. Given this context, and given that all three of his predecessors were ultimately exonerated after scathing battles with Dingell, it is unsurprising that Fisher might have been reluctant to square off with the prominent politician. Additionally, the contested existence of a gag order may have prevented him from speaking out. As Fisher and NSABP statistician Carol Redmond explained, "We were made aware that Dr. Poisson and St. Luc Hospital were under investigation by the OSI, and we were instructed not to discuss this matter except on a 'need-to-know' basis."[79] NCI officials disputed this claim at the first Dingell hearing, again leaving Fisher hanging in the wind.[80]

Nonetheless, the reluctant apologist persona that was forged in the clash between Dingell and Fisher emerges from stock characterizations of political, as opposed to technical, controversy and betrays the chasm between technical reasoning and the demands for public accountability. Because many of the public arguers were not inclined to buy into the technical reasoning that Poisson's falsifications did not alter the study's outcomes, Fisher's perceived reluctant apologetic stance proved nearly insurmountable. Glimmers of his rhetorical quandary are evident when, on the eve of his June 15 testimony, Fisher sat with his family in the Willard Hotel in Washington, DC. His Washington-based attorney, Joseph Onek, called to inform him of some concerns with his prepared testimony, which, consistent with congressional practice, had been circulated to Dingell staffers in advance.[81] "They said there isn't enough groveling," Onek told him.[82] In his public statement before the subcommittee, however, Fisher clearly declared that he accepted his "share of the responsibility for those administrative deficiencies that occurred" and conceded error, explaining that "perhaps my passionate attention to science overshadowed my administrative insight, and this was a mistake."[83] Fisher further affirmed that he "sincerely share[d] the subcommittee's concern regarding fraud in science" and offered deep regret at the "data falsification by a physician at one of the hospitals participating in the NSABP."[84]

Fisher's regret fell on deaf ears. As illuminated by Onek's telephone message concerning Fisher's prepared testimony and the unnamed Dingell staffer's assessment of its failures, Fisher's statement did not convince panel members of his sincerity. It failed because in the standards of a powerful congressman campaigning against big science, Fisher did not apologize enough, was not humble enough, and did not show the contrition that this powerful group thought was due.

Concerns about his April 13 testimony echoed this sentiment as well. One day before the April 13 oversight hearing, following a facsimile transmittal of Fisher's testimony to University of Pittsburgh lawyer Martin Michaelson, "word came back to Fisher that Michaelson didn't like anything about it."[85] According to Carpenter and Twedt, "Michaelson didn't think it had come close to accepting enough blame for what had happened."[86] After some discussion, Fisher's lawyers agreed with Michaelson's idea that Fisher should cite ill health and refuse to testify. Onek concurred, arguing, "'we just didn't know enough' about the allegations against the NSABP," and 'it didn't seem like a good time to do this.'"[87] According to Carpenter and Twedt, Michaelson "tried to soothe Fisher, suggesting at one point that he read poetry."[88] Michaelson's advice was to "keep quiet, don't say anything, and it will all blow over."[89] In retrospect, Michaelson's direction and characterization of the controversy missed the mark. As Carpenter and Twedt noted, the controversy did not blow over and in fact "would be listed as one of the top 10 stories of the year, according to the Associated Press."[90] Fisher's decision to take Michaelson's advice and not appear damaged his reputation further, especially when his healthy appearance at an oncology meeting several days later encouraged his congressional audience to attribute his absence to motives such as arrogance and disrespect.

Fisher's absence also provided the opportunity for other scientists representing the NCI to point the finger in his direction. For example, former NCI director Sam Broder testified in April that Fisher "did not respond to constructive criticism by NCI staff" and that he had not published a reanalysis of data when ordered to do so.[91] Broder apologized repeatedly, "we are very sorry," and assured Dingell's subcommittee that "errors will not happen again."[92] When Dingell noted that "top NCI officials have complained to the subcommittee staff that they could not even get Fisher to return their phone calls, let alone take any direction from the NCI," Broder did not correct his comment.[93] The *Cancer Letter* headline "NCI Apologizes for Mismanagement of NSABP; Says Fisher Resisted Criticism," provided a condensation of the problem: Fisher's absence had unwittingly conveyed a powerful message of arrogance, which resonated with earlier constructions of his persona.[94] Other institutional rhetors, sensing his scapegoating, and acting under institutional shields, further cordoned him off, as the *Cancer Letter* headlines "Univ. of Pittsburgh Distances Itself from Fisher" and "NSABP's Pink Sheet: Fisher's Control Had a Downside" revealed.[95]

Despite his scientific eminence, Fisher's rhetorical performance proved devastating. "Tragic for Bernard Fisher" announced the June 24, 1994, issue of the *Cancer Letter* under the subheading "Fisher Unable to Answer

Key Questions, Blames NCI."[96] One unnamed Dingell staffer told the *Post-Gazette* that "the real problem with Fisher's testimony" was that he "really couldn't come to grips with admitting the warts and wrinkles of the project."[97] "The hearings," noted George Goldberg, "were part inquiry, part hanging, with Fisher playing the role of captured varmint," chock full of "vitriol directed at Fisher."[98]

At the second hearing, Fisher attempted to persuade the Dingell subcommittee of his integrity and dogged devotion to research. The first six paragraphs of his forty-one-paragraph testimony tried to persuade others of his good intentions and commitment to science. By contrast to the other scientists who testified that day, who merely mentioned their current position, Fisher led with a description of his scientific accomplishments in order to stress his devotion to cancer research. He emphasized his passionate commitment to the study and treatment of breast cancer, underscoring that as a result of NSABP research, which he had chaired for thirty-five years, women could now choose to avoid disfiguring surgery.[99] He also enumerated the harms that befell him and others from the controversy. "The events arising out of the data falsification in Canada," he testified, "have been tragic for me, my colleagues, our families, and for all the women in this country." "Women," he concluded, "must not become victims of these events."[100]

Fisher's efforts to address Dingell's charges relied on three strategies in responding to Dingell's attack: denial, suggestion of harm, and ignorance of foreseeable consequences. First, Fisher rejected characterizations that he was less than honest in his actions and motives: "There was never any intent to hide information regarding the discovery of falsified data at St. Luc Hospital in Montreal, and I emphasize that. There was never any attempt by me or my associates to hide any information regarding the discovery of that information."[101] The characteristic use of passive voice so common in scientific prose nonetheless undercut Fisher's agency, as it sounded passive and ineffectual. Second, Fisher suggested that he was harmed by the allegations at the same time that he denied action and motive. "For 30 years," he explained, "the goal of the NSABP was to provide better information to patients and their physicians. The suggestion that we suppressed information is painful," he said, "We never attempted to hide any information. There could have been no conceivable reason to do so."[102] Here, Fisher attempted to demonstrate his credibility with direct appeals to reason. Finally, Fisher maintained that he did not anticipate the consequences of his communication strategy. "We didn't realize that the failure to publish our findings immediately would be misinterpreted by the public as an indication that we were concealing information," he testified. "Such a perception resulted in the unjustified concern that women with breast cancer were receiving inappropriate therapy."[103] "Let me emphasize this firmly," he stressed, "if our reanalyses had produced evidence that the conclusions of our studies were affected by the data alterations, we would have reported our findings immediately. Neither we, the NCI, the NIH, nor the OSI perceived that the Poisson falsifications had resulted in a public health problem."[104] Fisher thus appealed to technical, scientific grounds to make his case that Poisson's actions did not alter the lumpectomy study outcomes. However, that he was debating before Congress on terms of public argument meant many audience members, using public sphere reasoning, were unconvinced.

Fisher's testimony reveals a schism in the conceptions of the character of science between Fisher and his colleagues and many members of the public. In Fisher's view, science spoke for itself. The study's conclusions were unchanged, end of story. In the public's mind, any tainted data threatened the integrity of the entire enterprise. Thus, a gulf between perceptions of the scientific community and those of the public/Dingell regarding the seriousness of Poisson's actions cast doubt on the impact to the data. Fisher had trouble persuading the Dingell subcommittee that Poisson's falsifications, which Fisher noted were minimal and did not alter the outcome of the trial, did not put a taint on all NSABP research, and this suasive failure imperiled estimations of his integrity and trustworthiness. Although Fisher made the argument logically, as evidenced above, his faltering credibility undercut the effectiveness of that message. Moreover, his refusal to kowtow to Dingell forged the persona of a reluctant apologist on two levels: first, in a weaker sense in the opinion of his auditors, he refused to apologize sufficiently for his failures in handling the Poisson affair; second, in a deeper sense, he was a reluctant apologist for big science. He seemed to be saying, "The process works, let it alone, and let me do my important work unhindered by people who do not understand." Considering he was talking about taxpayer-funded research, many believed this position was inexcusable. Dingell's staffers thought Fisher's arrogance prevented him from assuming proper humility. According to Fackelmann, one Dingell staffer at the House hearings maintained that it was "'clear there was arrogance on Fisher's part.'"[105] Fackelmann opined, "Indeed, Fisher may have fallen victim to the same mind-set that felled Poisson—the belief that this work was so important, he could ignore the red tape of federal requirements."[106]

In 1997 twenty highly regarded European statistician-researchers, including Richard Doll, one of the founders of the modern clinical trial, published a *Controlled Clinical Trials* essay titled "The Trials of Dr. Bernard Fisher: A European Perspective on an American Episode." These authors penned an emphatic, imagined testimony that they would have given before Dingell's committee. It appeared in boldface in their text:

> It needs to be understood that randomization of a few slightly ineligible patients into a large clinical trial is a type of change that cannot introduce any material bias into the main results of that trial. What this means . . . is that the main types of alteration that Dr. Poisson made could not have introduced any material bias in the NSABP trial. So, even before the results were re-analyzed with and without his data and the results were submitted to the NCI, both NSABP and NCI officials knew that such changes couldn't make any material difference either way—and, of course, they didn't.[107]

Viewed from this perspective, Poisson's falsifications, though wrong, hardly damaged the study's conclusions. Yet assessments of the seriousness of Poisson's actions and the rightness of Fisher's oversight responses were not predestined. One strategy that Fisher did not employ effectively was to move the audience to see the misconduct as evidence of the self-correcting nature of science and as an aberration that did not taint NSABP research outcomes. In Fisher's view, and that of his European colleagues, the facts of the case meant it was obvious that the trial's conclusions still held up, that they still had integrity. In some segments of the public's view, as seen in the tearful testimony of Jill Sigal, however, any dishonesty cast doubt on the entire enterprise.

Science under the Bell Jar?

One interpretation of Fisher's silence and reluctant apologetic stance is that he misread the nature of his rhetorical situation because of his preference for insularity as a model of scientific inquiry. This misrecognition prevented him from responding appropriately according to those who interpreted the situation from a nonstatistical frame. Another view is that Fisher set himself up for attack by politicians by publicly calling them out. Despite his apparent success in persuading the NIH to fund the NSABP and persuading the medical community and American women in the value of his trials, Fisher's rhetoric reveals a strong preference for a separation of politics and science and a firm commitment to science's need to progress unbridled by bureaucracy. According to sources at the University of Pittsburgh, Fisher "often instructed students to avoid three things—'politics, process and publicity,'" a fact that appeared in the media at the height of the Datagate controversy.[108]

On May 17, 1993, nearly one full year before the public fury over Datagate would launch his downward spiral, Bernard Fisher stood before members of the American Society for Clinical Oncology (ASCO) to deliver his presidential address, titled "Thoughts from a Journey."[109] Fisher's speech was smattered with historical allusions and literary references as wide-ranging as the ancient Greek myth of Prometheus, aphorisms from Pittsburgh Steelers coach Bill Cowher, and the lines from Greek poet Konstantinos P. Kavafis's *Ithaca*.[110] Fisher devoted the first third of the speech to relaying his journey to the presidency of ASCO, which he called his "odyssey"—another gesture to the Ancients and to his struggles along the way—and which resulted in the "ridiculously low probability of [his] being on this podium as the 29th president" of the organization.[111] He began with a reference to his Promethean period, when he studied liver regeneration, and recounted the course of his career. Although a portion of the middle of the speech was devoted to chronicling some of the political battles ASCO had been involved in the year before, the thrust of the address was that the membership needed to steer clear of politics and embrace the concept of the clinical trial as the grand prospect of breast cancer research. Fisher identified "the second coming of the Periclean Age" as the time he became certain that clinical trials were the mechanism for determining the worth of new therapies. Indeed, he called the clinical trial "that wonderfully perfect device that I thought offered promise of restoring the Periclean Age."[112]

Fisher devoted much time in the final two-thirds of his ASCO speech promoting the ideal of clinical trials and admonishing his colleagues not to compromise clinical trials by succumbing to political battles. However, in attempting to unite the audience with the common vision of "preventing and curing cancer through scientific investigation, which includes both basic and clinical research," he demarcated scientists from three other dangerous species.[113] In the second section of the speech, subtitled "The Presidential Year," Fisher reviewed the turmoil that followed a unilateral split from the American Association of Cancer Researchers (AACR), with whom ASCO had been holding joint meetings since 1964. Fisher set up a division between oncologists and two other species: his in-elegant sounding "BAPs" and the public. He explained that "in my view, the widening gap between the clinician and the investigator could be a greater threat to the welfare of patients than are bureaucrats, administrators, and politicians (BAPs)."[114] Here, his brash voice heedlessly castigated both his clinician colleagues and those who funded his research. "As they become more and more subsumed by the BAPs' philosophy, clinicians get further away from science," he maintained, "where the hope for a progress and a cure for science resides."[115] He continued, "It can be guaranteed that BAPs will not become like clinicians, but, without the clinicians' allegiance to science, it cannot be guaranteed that the clinicians will not become indistinguishable from the BAPs."[116] Fisher may have been expressing ideas that the membership generally agreed with but that they may have been surprised he would air so publicly. Regardless of whether this speech resonated widely with members of his immediate audience, it is not difficult to see how it would trouble members of wider audiences, serving as an emblematic representation of scientific arrogance.

Fisher boldly continued to cordon off scientists from the rest of the world: "I still do not appreciate the virtue of public debate of scientific issues via sound bytes in the media, because this inappropriately shapes public opinion. That populist approach often results in the formation of paradigms of treatment similar to the way in which lobbyists influence legislators—another perfect example of antiscience."[117] These statements proved inflammatory when picked up by investigative journalists with good research skills at the height of the controversy, and may have even been interpreted by Dingell as Fisher's having throwing down the gauntlet.[118] Nonetheless, in affirming ASCO's importance and his place in it, Fisher was shoring up his place in oncological history. "As I complete this part of my journey that began at Stone House," he said, "I leave you with the admonition that, at no time in history has it ever been so important that all who are involved with cancer research and treatment maintain a united front."[119] In the dramatic conclusion of his speech, Fisher cautioned members that if they gave in to the pettiness of politics, they risked giving up scientific advancement with disastrous results: "More bluntly, there will result the end of a dream—the end of a dream for ASCO, the end of a dream for clinical trials, and perhaps even the end of a dream for biomedical research, one of this country's greatest treasures—and the new Periclean Age will need to await another time in history."[120]

While this warning may be understood within the context of battles internal to ASCO and AACR, Fisher's vision of an insular science appeared years before his 1993 ASCO speech in one of his *Cancer Research* charts, called "The Maelstrom of Research." This illustration depicted a clinical researcher besieged by attorneys, administrators, nurses, and patients. Fisher's commentary emphasized that researchers must avoid being drawn into the fray and must separate themselves from the undue influence of politicians, publics, and regulators to preserve their important work. Such was the view he expressed in his 1993 address. "I admit that, when I began my presidency, I was less than enthusiastic about ASCO's role in the public issues arena. I was convinced that such involvement could only distract ASCO from its primary mission of supporting research and education directed at curing and preventing cancer. I was fearful that the politics, process, and publicity associated with such efforts could achieve clonal dominance and destroy the host," he noted.[121]

> I soon learned, however, that in these chaotic times, one needs a mechanism to fend off the rascals who mine the road to progress with misguided causes they espouse with the fervor of zealots, or agendas that are totally self-serving. I believe that ASCO should be used as a bully-pulpit to express its position on selected public issues relevant to its major mission, which is the preservation and promotion of science. But ASCO should be forever vigilant that it is not so involved that it becomes—once again, to use the metaphor of *Animal Farm*— indistinguishable from those it opposes.[122]

Fisher then elaborated on two causes ASCO had taken up during his presidential year: (1) prodding Congress to increase the excise tax on cigarettes and (2) taking a stand against federal reimbursement of costs for patients enrolled in clinical trials. He explained, "It makes no sense that the National Cancer Institute (NCI) endorses trials while private insurance companies capriciously make decisions to deny payment for treatments used in those studies."[123]

This strict division that Fisher had tried to maintain between science and the BAPs would ultimately come back to haunt him. In the end, it put him at odds with the communities who could have supported him the most—his patients. As physician Drummond Rennie would later conclude: "The public places a good deal of confidence in us and supports workers, like Fisher and his colleagues, with tax money to find the best ways to deal with the diseases that are going to kill us. The worst aspect of this sorry story is not that Poisson committed misconduct but that the NSABP has seemed dilatory and secretive in answering to those who matter most—our patients."[124] Fisher's avowed aversion to politics and publicity (apart from seeking grant funding and publications) would undermine his case, for, as Rennie's statement illustrates, when working with public monies on treatments for a disease as prevalent as breast cancer, partnership with publics, rather than opposition to and separation from them, encourages support.

Fisher's post-Datagate rhetoric further confirmed his preference for an insular science. His 2000 Legacy Laureate address at the University of Pittsburgh was aptly titled "Insularity with Vision: Paradigm for Productivity in Science." Here, Fisher explicitly introduced a metaphor of insularity, a microscope in a bell jar, which sheds insight into why he was so reluctant to share news of Poisson's actions with various publics. Fisher recounted that when he had returned to his alma mater, the University of Pittsburgh, in 1952, he had "made it quite clear that [his] reason for an academic career was to conduct research," that he "really had absolutely no interest in the institutional politics, finance, administrative activities or even committee appointments."[125] Then one day, in the mid-1950s, Dr. William McElroy, former dean of the University of Pittsburgh's Medical School, gave Fisher an old microscope donated by the wife of a dead alumnus. According to Fisher, "That instrument became a metaphor of my life as a researcher, particularly when it was placed in a bell jar given to me by Norman Wolmark, one of my earlier disciples."[126] At this point in his narration, Fisher switched slides to project a picture of the microscope sealed in a bell jar, the glass shining against a white background. The photograph was crisp and austere. He continued to explain that microscopes function best when they are focused, and that focus comes from insularity, "his paradigm for productivity."[127]

Fisher's cultivated insularity, his microscope under a bell jar, forged before, during, and after the Datagate controversy, functioned as a microcosm for what many patients, cancer advocates, and colleagues believed was wrong in the first place: the silence on behalf of public officials with regard to information that could have affected the life-and-death treatment choices for women facing breast cancer. And that—coupled with perceptions of a gag order—was precisely the crux of the matter as to why Fisher did not vigorously go public with the news of Poisson's falsifications: he did not believe the falsifications altered the findings about lumpectomy. This, then, may have been Fisher's fundamental downfall: the misrecognition of the need to come clean to the public about the falsification and its meaning in the first place. Recall his stern pronouncement that "I still do not appreciate the virtue of public debate of scientific issues via sound bytes in the media, because this inappropriately shapes public opinion," which occurred one year before the public learned of Poisson's falsifications. Although in Fisher's mind there was no public health crisis, and thus no need for communication, in the view of many of his critics such communication was not only critical for patient well-being but it was also ethically required. "'Dr. Fisher was almost a hero in the 1970s,' said Cindy Pearson, program director of the National Women's Health Network. 'But my experience, and the experience of others over the last six years or so, is that Dr. Fisher also believes he's a hero, and he doesn't think he needs to listen to anyone else.'"[128]

In retrospect, Fisher's invocation of the Periclean Age in his ASCO speech seems ironically prescient. Not only was the Periclean Age known for intense cultural advancement, the growth of the Athenian population to 150,000, and the first foundering of democracy, but it also produced the best-known tragedies of ancient Greece, including Sophocles's *Oedipus the King*. In invoking the spirit of the Periclean dream, Fisher's speech foreshadowed another formation of his character to emerge during the latter part of the controversy: the tragic hero, a giant man brought down by some weakness or flaw in his character. As the fury, which reached a fevered pitch during the Dingell hearings, began to die down, the overall narrative of Datagate morphed from controversy to tragedy with Fisher now starring as tragic hero. Packed into this narrative was the implied argument that he was not responsible for wrongdoing, that he had been wronged and harmed by institutional forces beyond his control, and that he deserved sympathy and support rather than anger and blame.

When considered together, the overlapping but competing personae that coalesced early in Datagate emphasized a broader narrative that rendered Fisher a convenient scapegoat for what was arguably a systemic failure or even a sensationalized drama. Even many of those who wished Fisher had come forward sooner thought he had been unfairly targeted by Dingell. However, the focus on Fisher's character and the degree to which he lived up to the scientific ethos—as revolutionary, as beleaguered administrator, and in his reluctance to apologize, either for his own actions or for the scientific method—proved incompatible with the broader public's framing of the problem. Fisher's initial hesitance to speak also provided the occasion for others to control the dominant narrative, rendering him the agent responsible for lapses. By May 17, 1994, Fisher attacked constructions of himself as an "embattled doctor" with a powerful rhetoric of his own.[129] Although he did not attend the first Dingell hearing, Fisher appeared at the annual ASCO meeting, where he received a standing ovation.[130] In his address before ASCO, Fisher noted that his review of data showed that Poisson's falsification did not alter the findings. Still displaying defiance, reported the *Post-Gazette*, "He did not apologize for the snafu that allowed falsified data from 99 patients to be entered into the studies, and he did not directly address the delays in making the problems public."[131]

A May 20, 1994, *Pittsburgh Post-Gazette* editorial titled "Taking Advantage: The Competition Begins for Pitt's Prestigious Cancer Study" demonstrated the interaction of the persona of beleaguered bureaucrat with the reluctant apologist: "There's blood in the water and the sharks are coming out to feed," it read; "that's not a very attractive way to look at the altruistic world of medical research, but it appears to be the case."[132] The editorial explained that "the fact that Dr. Bernard Fisher, who headed the project at Pitt, was slow in publishing the new results and was perceived as arrogant and thus was not as compliant as he should have been has led to a firestorm of criticism."[133] Here, Fisher's publication delays are hitched not to technical reasons but to arrogance to cement a portrait of untrustworthiness.

Analyzing the personae that animated the controversy in the immediate months after it crescendoed assists in understanding why Datagate progressed as it did. The trifecta of swashbuckling revolutionary, reluctant apologist, and beleaguered bureaucrat maintained the focus on Fisher's actions rather than the perils of or ethical issues associated with clinical trial participation, its inclusion rules, and access to experimental treatments. Moreover, these initial three personae together are suggestive of how certain policy options targeted at individual transgressions reigned. While a small portion of the public discourse about this controversy focused on solutions that would more squarely address stakeholder concerns about Datagate, the vast majority scripted scientific stakeholders out of participation in public life. For instance, the persona of scientific revolutionary rested on the mythos of science as a sacred space reserved for cultural elites who could properly discern the meaning of clinical trials without public input, even when this science was conducted in the service of the public good. The reluctant apologist, with its sharp separation of publics and scientists, further accentuated this view. By contrast, the beleaguered bureaucrat as a scientific administrator betrayed the stunning weight of large-scale scientific projects in terms of staffing and management, but similarly did not guarantee participants a place at the table. It is therefore not surprising that the most loudly trumpeted resolutions and policy outcomes of the controversy focused not on communicating with affected stakeholders or on institutionalizing public participation in science that some stakeholders clamored for, but on enacting enhanced data monitoring and increased audits. Fisher's competing scientific personae, like those of Roger Poisson, thereby helped to shape perceptions of appropriate policy responses, for they embedded characters of science controversy into storylines that emphasized individual transgression and impurities, an account that will be taken up in chapter 4.

As emotions began to settle, Fisher's public suffering provided a rhetorical opening for recasting Fisher as a vindicated scientific visionary. The interacting constructions of Fisher as swashbuckling scientific revolutionary, as reluctant apologist, and as beleaguered administrator undercut his initial efforts to persuade his audience of his integrity. They also undermined, for a time, public faith in the outcomes of his science, and at the same time, they supported visions of science that scripted publics out of meaningful participation in research that directly affected them. The question remains: How did Fisher, and others, work to reverse perceptions of his character? The answer lies in the seeds of his pioneering revolutionary persona and in the growing sense, felt early and keenly by his supporters, that Fisher had suffered from Dingell's abuse of power.

CODA: SCIENTIFIC REVOLUTIONARY REDUX, BERNARD FISHER AS TRAGIC-HERO-TURNED-VINDICATED-VISIONARY

During the summer of 2002, the award-winning University of Pittsburgh Medical School alumni news magazine, *Pitt Med*, ran a feature titled "Bernard Fisher in Conversation." At the time of its publication, more than a decade had elapsed since the initial discovery of Roger Poisson's data falsification, and eight years had gone by since Congressman Dingell had called Fisher to testify before Congress. By all appearances, Bernard Fisher had been vindicated. Indeed, it is almost as if the controversy had been erased from the official record, even if it continued to live in the memories of medical community members who read the text when it arrived in their mailboxes in late July. Utterly silent with regard to the dramatic events of 1994, the feature made no reference to Datagate or to Fisher's schism with the University of Pittsburgh, instead focusing on Fisher's accomplishments and interlacing colorful autobiographical snippets from his "forty years at the University" (no mention of his forced resignation) with descriptions of his achievements and photographs from various stages in his career.[134]

The feature opened with a full-page snapshot of then-eighty-two-year-old Fisher seated at his desk. Bearded and smiling broadly, hands outstretched in a warm gesture, he welcomed the world. An apple sat prominently in the center foreground nestled among stacks of paperwork. Behind Fisher, on a bulletin board, hung papers neatly arranged in rows. The scene was vaguely academic, yet cozy, revealing the office of a busy man, a perception reinforced by the accompanying text: "Most of the horizontal space in his office is covered by papers and folders relating to his current projects." At the bottom of the page, in small blue type set against the black and white of the picture, read the caption: "It has been said that he has done more to improve the outlook for women with breast cancer than any other physician in the history of clinical research. And Bernard Fisher's studies had powerful implications for treatments of other cancers as well." Excerpts of interviewer Leah Kauffman's discussion with Fisher emphasized his commitment: "During my scientific life, I have been trying to make a contribution toward bettering the lives of women with breast cancer," Fisher said, enumerating the highlights: "Our 1998 report indicating, for the first time, that breast cancer could be prevented with tamoxifen was probably the capstone of my career"; "Certainly, in 1958, when I began this journey, the idea of using an agent to try to prevent breast cancer was … science fiction." The magnitude of Fisher's achievements, his challenge to Halstedian tenets, and his continued efforts to find treatments for breast cancer emerged as the central themes of the interview. From the photograph caption noting that Fisher had "done more to improve the outlook for women with breast cancer than any other physician in the history of clinical research" to phrases like "Fisher soon realized that members of the NSABP could help him test this new hypothesis," Kauffman's excerpted interview reinvigorated the persona of Fisher as scientific revolutionary but muted the swashbuckling register.[135]

Kauffman's introductory text placed Fisher's achievement in context by opening with the story of Betty Ford's much-publicized radical mastectomy in 1974, noting that while she was recovering from her surgery in Bethesda Naval Hospital, "Bernard Fisher, MD '43, of the University of Pittsburgh," was across the street at the NIH reporting "findings from studies that would have a profound effect on the treatment of breast cancer for the next 30 years." Fisher's several notable firsts comprised key points of emphasis. When commenting on his interest in the recent mammography controversy, for example, Fisher offered, "Incidentally, in 1974, I established, at Pitt, the first breast cancer detection center in Pittsburgh." After reviewing his career and offering his musings on clinical research, the interview ended with Fisher's observation that "it isn't over yet. I still have a full briefcase!" Thus, a portrait of an engaged visionary emerged. His past was significant in revolutionizing breast cancer treatment, his present was occupied with continuing studies, and his future was open to new discovery. Fisher was busy, but no longer beleaguered; the matter of Datagate was erased.[136]

How did the once "embattled" doctor arrive at this point? How did this vindication—and even this epideictic rhetoric extolling his accomplishments—come about? If Bernard Fisher were to tell the story, the answer would be simple: because he was innocent of wrongdoing and the world finally knew it. Indeed, this interpretation is one that many in the medical community and elsewhere are willing to offer. But for a rhetorician, the task that is more important than making absolutist judgments about guilt or innocence is explaining how language choices played a role in the transformation from swashbuckling scientific revolutionary, beleaguered bureaucrat, and reluctant apologist to the vindicated visionary.

During the summer of 1994, Fisher faced a dizzying onslaught of criticism that threatened his career, jeopardized his health, and tested him to his limits, sapping him of his vitality. By December the *Pittsburgh Post-Gazette* announced, "Fisher's Years of Achievement Crumble[d] Overnight."[137] Another opinion in the *Post-Gazette* noted that Fisher's "international acclaim" made his fall "all the more precipitous."[138] Similarly, Fisher is reported to have undergone a "staggering reversal of fortunes."[139] He was "the victim of nearly hysterical overreaction and political gamesmanship at its worst."[140] But finally, after a period of reticence and withdrawal, Fisher took action. On July 8, 1994, he filed suit against the University of Pittsburgh, its attorneys (including the Washington, DC, law firm Hogan and Hartson), and the National Cancer Institute. "Saying 'enough is enough,' Dr. Bernard Fisher charged yesterday that he had been made a scapegoat by the University of Pittsburgh and federal officials," announced the *Pittsburgh Post-Gazette* on July 13, 1994.[141] Thus, Fisher and his supporters crafted a tragic hero/scapegoat persona and catapulted it into the public sphere in a dazzling counterattack against institutional officials. "After months of declining to discuss his case extensively with journalists, Fisher appeared to launch a public relations offensive," reported the *Post-Gazette*'s Mackenzie Carpenter.[142] Fisher's legal action against the University of Pittsburgh and the federal government was sparked by his belief that the university and the NCI had denied him his constitutional right of due process when, alleging that Fisher had improperly managed a large, multisite clinical trial, they forced his resignation from NSABP chairmanship. He also sued the NCI for allowing improper labeling of all of his publications with the flag "scientific misconduct" when no such finding had been made. "I think the NCI overreacted when the whole thing happened and they began to put into effect all kinds of things that eventually led to my, as you put it, 'decapitation,'" Fisher told the *Post-Gazette*.[143] He filed the lawsuit "with a great deal of sadness and dismay," he explained, "because I've been part of the University of Pittsburgh family for forty years as a full-time academician."[144]

On July 15, three of six articles about Datagate appeared in the *Cancer Letter*'s table of contents: "Bernard Fisher Sues Univ. of Pittsburgh and Its Attorney," "Pittsburgh Broadens Inquiry to Include Lawrence Wickerham," and "100 NSABP Sites May Enroll Patients; Only One Trial Open."[145] The next week, "Pitt Inquiry Panel Proceedings Suspended, ORI to Take Over NSABP Investigation" was followed by "NSABP Executive Committee Is

Seeking Applications from Surgeons to Lead Group," and then by "ORI Takes Over Misconduct Inquiry of NSABP Officials," in late July.[146] August notices spread perceptions of his action further: "Fisher, NSABP Executive Committee, File Injunction Seeking Herberman's Removal," "Court Filing by Fisher, Board Attacks Interim NSABP Leadership," and "NSABP Executive Committee Joins Fisher's Suit against Pitt."[147] Fisher meanwhile had issued a statement saying that he was "saddened and reluctant to have to go to court to make a stand on behalf of all research scientists for fair treatment and due process from institutions like Pitt and from government bureaucracies like NCI."[148] Here, Fisher borrowed the collective ethos of the community of scientists. He verbally reconfigured his struggles with Pitt as a duel between all scientists and the bureaucracy in an attempt to remind others that he was not the sole target of the investigative zeal, but that *all* of science was in effect on trial.

Fisher continued to mount his challenge to his critics. In September 1994 he wrote a letter to NSABP investigators declaring, "I can no longer sit idly by and watch as political maneuvering and media frenzy not only continue to discredit NSABP studies but, by innuendo, all clinical trials, particularly those related to breast cancer."[149] Thus, he strengthened his narrative in which all of science, all of clinical research was under attack. He sought to relocate the issue away from his individual character to the context of science as a whole. Elsewhere, though, he did seek to preserve his own name, but often through referring to the NSABP as a collective. In a letter to the editor of the *Post-Gazette* in 1995, he sought to establish the integrity of the B-06 findings: "First, our original findings, as well as those from the re-analyses, indicate the lumpectomy followed by radiation therapy is effective, not only in women with small tumors, as you state, but in those with large tumors as well."[150] "We" and "our" are the pronouns here, not the first person seen in his efforts to craft a revolutionary persona. "The worth of breast preservation for the treatment of breast cancer has never been in doubt since we first reported the findings from the B-06 study in 1985," he insisted.[151] In addition, Fisher continued to present himself as a victim of government scapegoating: "Finally, the 'less-than-thorough auditing procedures' that you allude to, and the need 'to clean up (my) auditing act' was a false scenario created by Rep. John Dingell's staff and the NCI as another aspect of this bizarre political affair. Our auditing procedures were scapegoated to justify the actions taken by those groups."[152] These efforts to restore his name seemed to be taking hold in public discourse. The leitmotif of Fisher the victim of a zealous institutional witch hunt recurred. But conjoined with that refrain is the persistent suggestion that others are to blame for harming Fisher. His denials of wrongdoing were now coupled with attacks on the institutions that had until this point scapegoated him: "We assure you that any delay in publishing a paper presenting reanalyses of data was not a 'cover-up' since there was nothing to hide. Moreover, if the NCI and ORI had perceived that any such delay was harmful, they had full authority to 'get their message out' to physicians and the public."[153] The implication: I am not solely to blame here, folks. Moreover, Fisher charged that other parties needed to account for the harm done to science during this imbroglio. His September letter published in the *Cancer Letter* continued his attack on his accusers: "I remain troubled by the abrupt suspension of all NSABP clinical trials in progress and by the postponement in the development and start of the new studies. These events could affect the lives of thousands of breast cancer patients in years to come. I believe this was a dangerous and ill-advised action for which there must be accountability."[154]

Even the responses to Fisher's lawsuit that decried it as a recuperative strategy echoed Fisher's tragic hero persona. "It is easy to identify with Dr. Bernard Fisher's utterly human impulse to sue the University of Pittsburgh in an attempt to get his job back and, in effect, clear his name. But while we sympathize, we wish he hadn't done it," began an unsigned July 22 editorial in the *Pittsburgh Post-Gazette*. "Although it is understandable that, after making such monumental contributions to medicine and science, Dr. Fisher would rather not see his career end as it did," his lawsuit "is likely merely to dissipate his energies and dilute his message" and "ultimately, may be as ill-conceived as the stonewalling strategy Pitt and its lawyers originally advised Dr. Fisher to follow." The editorial stated: "Dr. Fisher may have been responsible for some lax administrative oversight; for unnecessary delay in reporting his re-analysis; and for continuing to publish articles that didn't exclude the data even after he knew it was tainted. But any such failings—and he does not concede that they are problems—fade into insignificance next to the phenomenally important work he has done." "It is also possible that baser political and personality disputes played a part in creating this overheated atmosphere," the editorial admitted. Fisher "is not blameless in the controversy that has clouded the close of his brilliant career," the editorial opined prematurely, but "his removal may have been the unavoidable cost of restoring confidence in the study in the wake of the controversy or it may have a pound of political flesh."[155] From the fall from greatness and a devastating personality flaw to the sense that Fisher's suffering was unavoidable, the elements of tragedy conjoined at a high cost to Fisher.

Accounts of the tragic nature of Fisher's fall appeared in newsletters, newspapers, and professional journals. For instance, the June 24, 1994,

Cancer Letter described Fisher's rocky testimony at the Dingell hearing as "tragic."[156] Barbara Seltman, then executive director of the Cancer Support Network in Pittsburgh's Shadyside neighborhood, dubbed the controversy an "unfair and tragic episode in the life of Dr. Fisher."[157] Seltman explained that "for those of us who have survived the fires of cancer, it behooves us to be advocates of the Dr. Bernard Fishers of the world, the selfless pioneers who pave the way for the medicine of the future."[158] In these accounts Fisher thus becomes a brave hero unjustly brought down. In 1997 twenty European authors collaborated on an article asking what all the American fuss was about regarding Datagate. These authors wholeheartedly endorsed Fisher. "To those of us a few thousand miles away from America, this whole Kafkaesque episode seems absurd, but also nasty."[159]

If tragedy, in both the Aristotelian and the popular sense, involves a fall, then Datagate provided immense fodder for the construction of Fisher as tragic hero. An editorial in the *Post-Gazette* noted that Fisher's "international acclaim" made his fall "all the more precipitous."[160] Similarly, Fisher is said to have undergone a "staggering reversal of fortunes."[161] He was "the victim of nearly hysterical overreaction and political gamesmanship at its worst."[162] As onlookers watched the spectacle of a great man careening down from empyrean heights to mortal realms, many were drawn to participate in the swirl of epideictic rhetoric. Former patients and other supporters rushed to Fisher's defense. Albert Smolover of Squirrel Hill opined, "Our city fathers should be busy defending Pitt and Fisher" in a May 29 letter to the editor. "We seem to be living in a time when mean-spirited people, headline-hunting politicians and misguided or irresponsible media find it necessary to destroy the reputations of institutions as well as individuals, including President Clinton, Anita Hill, and Dr. Fisher."[163] Mary Ann King of Brighton Heights, Pennsylvania, wrote a two-hundred-word letter to the editor recollecting the time she sat on an examining table in Fisher's office as a thirty-five-year-old mother of two young children ten years before: "Knowing of Dr. Fisher's expertise, reputation, professionalism, and dedication to women's health sustained me as I faced many difficult decisions and an uncertain future."[164] "Cheers to Dr. Bernard Fisher for the strength and tenaciousness he displayed in his long struggle to restore his reputation and good name," she wrote, "something I never for a moment doubted."[165]

Viewed from this perspective, Fisher's stature made him a suitable character for a tragic frame. Thus, the revolutionary scientist we met earlier was well poised to star as tragic hero in later events, especially if this revolutionary had a reputation for being arrogant. Many affirmed the harm the scandal had on a giant like Fisher, even early in the controversy. For instance, NSABP member Robert Cooper from Bowman Gray Medical School noted that "this is absolutely devastating to one of our most prestigious clinical trialists."[166] Lewis Kuller, then head of Pitt's epidemiology department, later maintained that there were few higher figures one could attack: "if you can go after people the quality of Bernie Fisher, you can go after anyone."[167] Yet Fisher was constructed as "good," even "great," but not too good, and certainly not entirely perfect. Dr. Samuel Hellman of the University of Chicago told the *New York Times,* "Bernie made some mistakes and NCI made some mistakes, but I would not like to see him be the fall guy."[168] Dr. Susan M. Love, a nationally renowned breast cancer doctor, noted in the *Los Angeles Times:* "It's sad. Fisher has been a very important figure. He's really been on the forefront of trying to figure out new ways of treating breast cancer. He's one of the few creative thinkers that we have, and I don't think he's actually done anything terrible."[169] Nonetheless, Love did go on to say, "I think that he should have released the information sooner, but my guess is that he probably didn't think it would make any difference. And he was right. It didn't."[170]

Even before Datagate, Fisher constructed himself as a man persecuted by others. This thread runs through much of his biographical rhetoric both before and after the controversy. During his rise to the status of revolutionary scientist, Fisher faced a number of obstacles, including others' hesitance to accept his ideas, delayed publication of his research findings, and political infighting. Fisher relied on these events as an argumentative resource for constructing himself as someone persistently attacked by others. The effect of this strategy is that it magnified the scope of his success: not only is he a revolutionary because of his ideas, but he is a martyr who achieved their actualization at great personal cost and in the face of enormous obstacles. "It seems that nothing is quite so effective in eliciting the meanness of the human spirit as clinical trials' research," Fisher told the ASCO membership in 1993, when he referenced criticisms of his efforts over the years.[171] Similar to Odysseus, to whom his description "odyssey" gestures, Fisher highlighted a number of battles along his journey. In 2002 he alluded to his view that others' "prejudice" allowed them to jaundice his successes. "Unfortunately, after four decades of investigation, I've recognized that discovery is not always triumphant. There's a sign right there. *[He points to the cabinet across the room, papered with his own maxims.]* It says, 'I speak, I write, others tell you what I mean. Prejudice can alter perception more profoundly than hallucinogens.'"[172] By indexing his suffering brought about by the unfair treatment of others, Fisher is able to solidify his tragic hero status long after the controversy had been formally resolved.

During the controversy itself, Fisher repeatedly reminded others of the harms he had suffered as Datagate unfolded. "The events arising out of the data falsification in Canada have been tragic for me, my colleagues, our families, and for all the women in this country" he announced in the opening of his June apologia before Dingell.[173] By continually recounting his struggles, Fisher could evoke the emotions of pity and fear, the two emotions Aristotle identified as central to tragedy. Eight weeks after Crewdson's initial report, at the May 16, 1994, ASCO meeting in Dallas, Fisher spoke before ASCO's plenary session in Dallas. He received standing ovations before and after his address when he described how "my life and that of my associates and that of the NSABP precipitously began to unravel."[174] He added, "We and our families are completely devastated as a result of the recent events."[175]

By late 1994 the initial public outcry was settling down. The *Pittsburgh Post-Gazette* presented a series of articles that not only humanized Fisher but also crafted a picture of him as a man of character who had suffered greatly. One of them relied heavily on emotional appeals, by describing him as dispirited and blocked from completing his lifework:

> He waits for the completion of a federal investigation into studies he published. He waits for the resolution of his lawsuit against the University of Pittsburgh. He waits, most of all, for vindication.
>
> At 76 years old, with his spirits flagging and his legal bills mounting, he feels precious time slipping away. The pre-eminent breast cancer researcher is cut off from the important work that has consumed his life.[176]

Such passages evoked pity for Fisher, portrayed as hardworking and tireless in the face of Dingell's investigative zeal. "Each day, he still goes to work at his old offices in the University of Pittsburgh's Scaife Hall," the article continued. "But instead of analyzing data that might lead to medical advances, Fisher confers with lawyers, writes defenses of his actions and takes calls from colleagues expressing sympathy."[177] Thus, the great scientist is prevented from continuing his life-saving discoveries and instead forced to contend with the comparatively trivial details of restoring his image and clearing his name. Even further, the man "renowned for his self-assurance" had "fallen into a deep depression."[178] The ordeal "'was a devastating thing for me,'" he said.[179] The focus on the personal details of how Fisher's everyday life were affected by the controversy personalized his suffering, rendering it more potent for readers. Who could resist feeling sorry for Fisher, the "embattled doctor?"[180]

Those who knew him might even have been affected more than the casual reader, however. "Cancer researchers around the country said they were saddened by the controversy surrounding Fisher, one of the founders of NSABP, who is widely respected for having designed and led innovative studies that changed the standard treatment for breast cancer," claimed the *Cancer Letter* with its usual flair.[181] The oncology newsletter, with its weekly installments of Fisher's follies, worked in two contradictory ways. It assisted with assignment of blame to Fisher as beleaguered bureaucrat so caught up with the breast cancer prevention trial that he could not attend to routine audits, but it simultaneously worked to promote a sense of concern for his suffering that also encouraged sympathy and solidarity. The table of contents from the June 24 *Cancer Letter*, for example, furthered the image of an "embattled" man. It includes the following list of articles: "University of Pittsburgh Distances Itself from Fisher," "Zeneca Says NSABP Was Tardy in Reporting Uterine Cancer Deaths," "A Transcript: What Fisher Knew, When Did He Know," "NSABP's Pink Sheet: Fisher's Control Had a Downside, Review Said," and a last item announcing available research funds.[182] While it is clear in each of these items that Fisher is being blamed for negative events, the fusillade of invective also functioned to elicit support for a man who appeared to be fighting against institutions with greater resources and power than any one man could possibly counter.

Colleagues, citizens, and patients paying attention to the coverage were invited to feel fear as a result of what was happening to Fisher as well. "If a scientist of the stature and accomplishment of Dr. Fisher can be publicly humiliated and his career destroyed—if, in effect, he can be given the death penalty for a serious traffic violation—then the rest of the research community has legitimate cause for concern," noted the *Pittsburgh Post-Gazette*.[183] "People are absolutely terrified of this Dingell business," explained one researcher.[184] The emotions elicited by the public ventilation of the tribulations of Fisher and the "beleaguered breast cancer project" involved onlookers in an experience of the entertainment functions of tragedy as spectacle, for who could not be drawn into the drama?

As an apologetic strategy, emphasizing Fisher's suffering and rendering Fisher himself a victim shifted the locus of moral responsibility away from Fisher onto others. "It's almost as if the National Cancer Institute is afraid that somebody is going to blame them for something, so they're blaming someone else," Dr. Walter Lawrence Jr. noted.[185] Lawrence maintained during Datagate that Fisher's "intellectual honesty and his interest in pursuing things above board have always been so clear cut. It feels as if the various parts of government are trying to make a goat out of him."[186] Hence, he forged an interpretation of events in which Fisher was the victim of institutional rhetors trying to pass the buck, a view that Fisher himself spread. If Fisher was, as the *Post-Gazette* proffered, a "victim of nearly hysterical overreaction and political gamesmanship at its worst," then surely he was not at fault.[187] Moreover, he would deserve support, pity, and sympathy for his forbearance.

Yet if Fisher is rendered an innocent victim, then innocence's dialectical counterpart, guilt, must appear somewhere else in the narrative. In making himself a goat, and hence a victim, Fisher and those who shared this view turned the blame on Dingell and administrative officials at the University of Pittsburgh and NCI. Other members of the medical community also offered accounts of the incident that absolved Fisher and blamed institutional agents for inappropriately scapegoating Fisher. In crafting an imaginary testimony they would have given to Dingell, twenty European investigators placed the blame on NCI and the University of Pittsburgh. They wrote:

> In an ideal world, the [1994] director of the U.S. NCI and his colleagues should have helped defend those running the NSABP by explaining to the press that there never could have been any scientific or clinical urgency in republishing any of those trials. (At that time, the ORI was telling the press that "we knew we were not facing a public health disaster.") Instead, perhaps because NCI members were going to be grilled by Congressman Dingell and his committee, the NCI directorate did the opposite: the NCI directorate instructed the University of Pittsburgh to remove Dr. Fisher from the chairmanship of the NSABP and to halt recruitment into the NSABP trials, and the university went ahead and did it. By conventional standards of academic integrity, the NCI shouldn't have given this order and, even if they did, the university should have refused it. But there's not much point in looking for a new set of supposed villains by trying to work out which people at the NCI and at the University of Pittsburgh behaved inappropriately. Indeed, one could even argue that if the NCI knew that they faced large budget cuts from Congress unless they found a "guilty person" to fire, then they had to fire somebody, even if they knew that nobody was really guilty.[188]

In December 1994 the *Pittsburgh Post-Gazette* reported that "on a bulletin board outside Fisher's office in Scaife Hall at the University of Pittsburgh, a *New York Times* profile of Dingell is posted, with one sentence underlined and marked with yellow highlighter. " 'To his critics, though,' the sentence reads, 'the 68-year-old Dingell was a bully; mean-spirited, vindictive and power-hungry.' "[189]

No doubt, Bernard Fisher—like David Baltimore, Bernadine Healy, David Gallo, and other scientists summoned to Congress before him— experienced this sentiment to be true. Fisher faced formidable opponents and powerful institutional forces, and yet he was not without rhetorical resources. Although emerging from Dingell's room in the Rayburn Building entirely unscathed was impossible, having prevented or minimized such an event in the first place through a well-crafted response to the *Chicago Tribune*'s initial report or preemptive notification to regulatory agencies might have assuaged a few critics or won a few supporters. In the end, the decision to remain silent on the controversy arguably proved to be Fisher's largest rhetorical miscalculation.

Eventually, however, the tide turned. On April 27, 1997, Fisher announced the withdrawal of his lawsuit against the University of Pittsburgh and the U.S. government. The terms of the settlement dictated that Fisher would receive apologies from both the university and the NCI, which agreed to pay a nearly three-million-dollar settlement, three hundred thousand dollars of which would come from NCI. The university's formal statement expressed "sincere regret at any harm or public embarrassment that Dr. Fisher sustained," underscoring that "at no time was Dr. Fisher found to have engaged in any scientific or ethical misconduct."[190] Finally, having been formally cleared of wrongdoing by the ORI and having received apologies and a settlement, he could emphasize his mistreatment even more boldly. A 1997 press release hammered the point:

> Dr. Fisher is relieved that his research has been vindicated and that he and his colleagues have been cleared of scientific misconduct. However, the damage that has been done to them by this baseless investigation has been extensive. Even more important, however, is the damage that has been done to science, scientists, cancer research, and the breast cancer patients and their families whose fears were so shamelessly inflamed for political purposes. The millions of taxpayer dollars that were spent for this purpose would have been far better spent in the pursuit of a cure for breast cancer.[191]

That Fisher's message already seemed to be taking hold is evident in the descriptions of him that appeared in the newspapers.[192] By 1996 Fisher was once again named "an acclaimed breast cancer researcher" rather than an "ousted chair" or "embattled researcher," even if he did not have final resolution on his legal battles or the ORI investigation against him.[193]

In 2000 Fisher drew a standing ovation after he vigorously insisted on his blamelessness during his Legacy Laureate speech, delivered at the University of Pittsburgh Medical Grand Rounds. Here, Fisher publicly proclaimed his innocence and altogether dismissed ideas that his judgment during Datagate had been clouded. "Did this [invitation to speak] have to do with redemption?" he asked the assembled audience? "I doubted that," he opined, "since redemption implies forgiveness for a misdeed, and since none was committed, that certainly shouldn't be the reason." He continued: "Was this invitation related to my resurrection? If that was the case, it was already too late, because I had been resurrected."[194] He then gestured toward the screen and projected a photograph of himself with a spotlight framing his head against a blue stage curtain. "For some reason, this halo got stuck on me," he said with a wry smile. The audience chuckled lightly. "So, that was that." Having overcome adversity, Fisher summarily rejected his treatment during the painful days of Datagate. He was thus redeemed, hints of wrongdoing were erased, and his status as a hero was magnified and secured.

After taking the stage, Fisher reviewed his journey to his present station in life with reference to his intersection with significant cancer research developments. He underscored changes in understanding regarding tumor biology, discussed the role of hormones in spurring cancer growth, and reviewed advances in various treatment modalities. In the final minutes of his address, he cryptically revisited the unfortunate events surrounding B-06. "In March 1994," he said, "the ultimate disaster in my career took place when politics interfaced with science, and my insularity was destroyed, that wonderful haven of nearly forty years, my bell jar at 914 Scaife Hall was precipitously shattered and as a result my microscope was exposed to the elements, thus completely destroying its focus."[195]

Fisher's metaphor of the microscope under the bell jar encapsulated his paradigm for productivity in science—scientists, he implicitly argued, require isolation and protection from political interference.[196] This view, as we discovered earlier in this chapter, undermined, for a time, his efforts at reputational rehabilitation. However, Fisher soon moved on from this idea, continuing, "Dr. Levine, once again, I am truly grateful to you for this invitation." The audience waited. Would he say no more? Almost sensing their unrest, Fisher admonished, "There is one more slide; don't go away." He shifted and began speaking anew in what has been described as his characteristically "gravelly" voice: "I do confess, however, to having the same feelings that Galileo so eloquently expressed in 1621." And so he pulled up a black Power Point slide, from which he read aloud, underscoring the words with a red laser pointer:

> "I have never understood, Your Excellency, why it is that every one of the studies I have published in order to please or to serve other people has aroused in some men a certain perverse urge to detract, steal, or deprecate that modicum of merit which I thought I had earned, if not for my work, at least for its intention" (Galileo, 1621).

"Thank you," he concluded. Realizing that was all he would say, the audience, including the author of this book, rose to its feet. And thus, labeled a Legacy Laureate by invitation and confirmed by standing ovation, Fisher rhetorically recast his role during Datagate to that of persecuted genius. Emblematically linking himself to the scientific icon of political harassment par excellence, Fisher scripted himself as part of a drama in which powerful interests had unsuccessfully tried to discredit his paradigm-shaping life's work. No longer operating under the taint of Datagate, Fisher triumphantly returned to Scaife Hall, the original scene of his decades-long NSABP research, and stood tall in the very building from which he had been unceremoniously excommunicated in the spring of 1994.

Rhetorician Edward P. J. Corbett once asked, "What perversity is there in the human psyche that makes us enjoy the spectacle of human beings desperately trying to answer the charges leveled against them?" "Maybe secretly," he mused, "we say to ourselves, 'Ah, there but for the grace of God go I.' We soon learn that not only can sticks and stones break our bones, but words can break them too."[197] The interacting constructions of Fisher as swashbuckling revolutionary, reluctant apologist, and beleaguered bureaucrat undercut for a time his efforts to persuade his audience of his integrity, yet they also provided the seeds for his redemption and symbolic reconfiguration as a tragic-hero-turned-vindicated-visionary.

The skirmishes over the character of Bernard Fisher, what his character meant for the NSABP, and how it affected the findings of one of the twentieth century's most important breast cancer studies reveal the broader antimonies between science, publics, and politicians, and explain how policy solutions that failed to address the overall issues concerning patient participation in science went largely untapped. The focus on Fisher's actions encouraged discussion that largely accepted the status quo of clinical trials, leaving some of the broader political topics concerning patient participation in clinical trial research unexamined. In the battles between Fisher and the "BAPs," we discover characterizations that divulge the underlying dilemmas of big science. Analysis of the competing characterizations of Fisher during Datagate thus registers the underlying dwelling place of science as one that was largely separated from public participation, even when its findings would directly bear on the health and well-being of particular publics. The mythic revolutionary churned scientific change solo, the beleaguered bureaucrat made an ill-fated decision that tainted data was not worth public notification, and the reluctant apologist failed to overcome the gap between publics and scientists with adequate contrition. Yet the tragic-hero-turned-vindicated-visionary recirculated themes from the revolutionary persona, casting Fisher in a righteous light as a man who had been unjustly persecuted by politicians for their personal gain.

These dueling characterizations thus disclose the tensions and challenges inherent in the ethos, the dwelling place, the underlying shape and norms of contemporary biomedical science. They reveal the political struggles of scientists aiming to preserve jurisdiction over their knowledge-producing domain. The conflict evidences the desire to preserve for the conduct of science a sacred and purified space freed from public infringement at the same time they expose this vision as untenable. Science-based controversies, and the characterizations that accompany and sustain them, therefore rely on, shape, extend, and reconfigure tacit understandings of who the scientist is and what his or her relationships are to the various stakeholders whose lives and well-being are thoroughly and deeply reliant on its practices and outcomes. These emergent personae reveal as much about our collective desires and anxieties about science as they do about the particular scientists who find themselves in the crossfire of science-based controversy.

4

Fighting for a Place at the Table

Women as Consumers, Partners, and Subjects of Science—and the "Dark Knight" Who Tried to "Protect" Them

On April 13, 1994, the voices of cancer patients and women's health advocates reverberated through Rayburn Hall as they testified during Congressman Dingell's hearing on "scientific misconduct in breast cancer research."[1] Although the panels featured a powerful cast of cancer coalition members and congresswomen, research oversight officials and representatives of Big Pharma, the star of the show was Jill Lea Sigal, a thirty-two-year-old cancer survivor whose poignant testimony was met with hushed silence before it captivated evening news viewers and recirculated through North American newspapers and medical publications.[2] "How many women must now wonder, as I do every day, if they will die because they may have made the wrong decision?" she asked. "How many women, Mr. Chairman, will die?"[3] Although this haunting question captured media fancy by emphasizing the existential terror facing women with cancer, the words of other women raised broader political questions about the extent of women's participation in federally funded research. For instance, Fran Visco, president of the National Breast Cancer Coalition (NBCC), used her testimony to chastise scientists' apparent disregard for cancer patients and survivors who first learned of problems with NSABP lumpectomy data when they had read the *New York Times*. Visco aligned herself with the 2.6 million women living with breast cancer, marking breast cancer survivors as "everyone": "We are lawyers, scientists, Members of Congress, teachers, homemakers, mothers, daughters," she explained. "We are, by and large, a medically sophisticated vocal group who live day in and day out with the threat, the fear and the pain of breast cancer." Speaking on behalf of this large and formidable group, Visco reminded listeners that "the anxiety and fear with which we live daily has been exacerbated by a barrage of events," including especially "the fundamental flaw in the systems that are supposed to protect us." She implored Congress and the scientific community to recognize that cancer advocates deserved a "place at the table."[4]

As both Sigal and Visco so resoundingly underscored, women affected by NSABP research hailed from all walks of life and occupied varying subject positions and relationships to cancer advocacy. Some were patients trying to protect the reputations of their beloved, life-saving surgeons; some were study participants incensed by researchers' paternal silence about problems with treatment data; some were activists fighting for increased participation in research and attention to the environmental causes of cancer; some were lifelong physicians striving for conceptual clarity—and many cut across several of these groups.[5] While a portion of women who spoke out during Datagate deemed the scandal an abomination, others could not comprehend why their compatriots were surprised or confused. Although their voices formed a powerful core of complaints, in the decade before blogs and message boards came to dominate public life, much of the vernacular rhetoric about Datagate—the everyday communication that occurred around water coolers, over phone lines, or in support groups—is lost to history, so one of the challenges I faced in this study was to represent women's concerns without replicating the silencing of, or the speaking for, women that occurred as the controversy progressed. Thus, against the backdrop of the official voices of the NCI and NSABP, which sought publicly to reassure women that lumpectomy was still safe, in this chapter I seek to recover and then to analyze women's voices as they appeared in mass media accounts, interviews, editorials, letters to the editor, books, and congressional testimony. The news of Poisson's treachery and Fisher's silence was, for many women, a call to speak and act—and act they did, in remarkably textured local and national showings. The growing chorus of other women who spoke out during the controversy testifies to the slipperiness of trust in biomedical research, wherein researchers and those who benefit from research are separated by a chasm of noncommunication. Their voices reveal the dilemmas of stakeholder exclusion from and inclusion in the research process, illuminating how the scientific endeavor is helped and hindered by more voices. But these voices also provide the opportunity to understand what happened at a moment when women felt compelled to contribute to the broader controversy over research that affected their lives. These voices—and those who spoke for them—form the primary focus of this chapter.

Because women entangled longer-term collective political struggles for participation in cancer research with the more immediate and intimate goal of assessing what Poisson's actions meant for individual treatment decisions, their speech during Datagate reveals the contradictions of contemporary breast cancer research. It both articulates and obscures the persistence of the borders, boundaries, and connecting walls between those whose lives are affected by research and those who conduct it; the undeniable power of biomedicine and its susceptibility to wider social influences; and the simultaneously destructive and productive power of technical communication to soothe or alarm patients facing threats to their health and well-being. Women's speech during Datagate further fuses the desire to be part of science with the emplacement of women outside of science and forms powerful stories about the promises and perils of being citizens, scientists, breast cancer patients, survivors, activists, and politicians who try to wrestle with scientific claims in a highly politicized and deeply uncertain atmosphere. Representative Patricia Schroeder summed up the situation when she noted that "women have very little trust right now because their research has been compromised."[6]

Seen from this perspective, Datagate can be understood as a struggle for ownership, wherein breast cancer patients, pharmaceutical researchers, oversight officials, scientists, and advocacy groups attempted to gain control of the terms of public debate and discussion.[7] A place at the table, the capacity to exert influence over the scientific peer review and agenda-setting processes, is one of the hardest-fought demands of health advocacy groups. Yet responses to the controversy often positioned women and health advocates outside that process by relegating them into consumer roles. In this way, the analysis of characterization that animates this chapter has implications for debates about *agency,* the ability for one's speech and action to make a difference, and for *representation,* the ability to speak and act for oneself or another. As we shall see, such matters of agency and representation were complicated in the Datagate scandal because so many participants spoke on behalf of the women of this country. Indeed, from Bernard Fisher to John Dingell, from Roger Poisson to Fran Visco and Jill Sigal, many persons clamored to speak for the "women of this nation." The rhetorical power of such testimony derived from the shared frame of women as having been harmed by the deceptions of Datagate. A closer inspection of the contours of this characterization, however, uncovers a more complicated tangle of colliding interests, conflicting motives, and diverse rhetorical strategies. Taken together, these colliding interests and tangled motives expose the dilemmas of public exclusion from and inclusion in the research process and policymaking arenas.

After offering a brief history of women's participation in breast cancer advocacy during the twentieth century, this chapter considers the dilemmas of representation of women's characters, of speech by, for, and on behalf of women during Datagate. When women speak on behalf of a collective before the ministers of science and government, whose voices are privileged? Which women speak for all women? On the issues associated with speaking for others, philosopher Linda Alcoff has noted that "who is speaking, who is spoken of, and who listens is a result, as well as an act, of political struggle."[8] "Simply put, the discursive context is a political arena," she explained, "to the extent that this context bears on meaning, and meaning is in some sense the object of truth, we cannot make an epistemic evaluation of the claim without simultaneously assessing the politics of the situation."[9] Heeding Alcoff's implicit call to assess the politics of who is speaking, this chapter addresses three key questions: What are the dilemmas that women faced when trying to make sense of Datagate? What major representations of women emerged during the controversy, and did these characterizations unwittingly reproduce divisions between science and stakeholders? How did these characters influence the progression of the case in ways that structured the health-care choices available to patients and providers? Ultimately, I argue that three dominant characterizations—the knowledge consumer, the subject of science, and the knowledge partner—encapsulate representations of women and other advocates' roles during Datagate. Unlike the personae that animated the previous chapters, which were tied to specific individuals, these personae are composites that reflect "the spirit or group character of a broader community of speakers."[10] Given the relative newness of women's efforts to participate in breast cancer research, it is not surprising that these cultural types are more blended, less fine-grained, and less biographically focused than the personae of Fisher and Poisson, because they are condensed representations of larger struggles to secure representation and participation in biomedical research. They nonetheless tended to draw on traditional gender roles and political frames as they condemned the silence on the part of the scientific community. However, each composite contains different possibilities for political representation in science, and they therefore disclose alternative visions of the place of science in public life.

WOMEN'S PARTICIPATION IN BREAST CANCER
CAUSES AND THE RISE OF CANCER ADVOCACY

By now it is a truism to say that for much of the twentieth century, women's breasts—those embodied, erotically electrified emblems of both physical longing and maternal care—remained under the medical care of men. Decisions made about cancer treatment tended to come from doctors, husbands, and male relatives, and often occurred in the hushed tones of private spaces. However, despite concealment of dominant surgical treatments and decision making within the private realm, the twentieth century also ushered in a long arc of breast cancer activism in which women played an increasingly vocal and prominent role. This explains why watching the apparent erosion of hard-won political battles as signified by the tardy disclosure of Datagate problems must have felt to some women like a knife in the back.

Women's participation in breast cancer advocacy rose along with their enhanced political status over the course of the twentieth century. Early efforts at promoting awareness involved several prominent wealthy women and their financiers but retained male dominance in leadership positions. The formation of the American Society for the Control of Cancer (ASCC) in 1913 is a case in point. Although the organization was founded by the affluent Mrs. Elsie Mead, and later transformed into the American Cancer Society (ACS) in 1946 by Mary Lasker, its leadership tended toward male domination; women performed support roles. The ACS Web site credits not Mead but "15 prominent physicians and business leaders in New York City" with its founding, boasting that "it was one of the most remarkable moments in the history of public health."[11] Doctors and surgeons formed the core of membership, although starting in 1936, ASCC, at the suggestion of field representative Marjorie G. Illig, chair of the General Federation of Women's Clubs Committee on Public Health, formed a volunteer Women's Field Army.[12] Garbed in khaki uniforms, women of the Field Army took to the streets to raise money and awareness. Clarence Little, then managing director of ASCC, noted that "in 1935 there were 15,000 people active in cancer control throughout the United States. At the close of 1938, there were ten times that number," largely because of the efforts of the Women's Field Army.[13] While the early years may have been characterized by grassroots organizing and modest educational efforts, in recent years the ACS has been criticized for being too "establishment" as it grew to become the largest private charity in the United States, boasting more than two million volunteers.[14] Thus, the success of the ACS transformed the organization into a bustling bureaucracy capable of influencing the contours of breast cancer education and treatment on a national scale.

In the meantime, feminist stirrings of the 1960s paved the way for collective action in the 1970s. In 1973 the Boston Women's Collective published *Our Bodies, Ourselves*. Two years later, Rose Kushner's *Breast Cancer: A Personal History and Investigative Report* appeared, and Kushner started the Breast Cancer Advisory Center (BCAC), a help and information hotline. Three years later, the seeds for the first breast cancer support hotline were sown in Chicago when Mimi Kaplan and Ann Marcou, two breast cancer survivors, started Y-ME. Thus, if the first wave of breast cancer activism comprised philanthropic efforts designed to improve awareness and promote surgery, the second wave—which dovetailed with the rise of feminism—increasingly featured women's public narratives, consciousness raising, and social support. Shattering decades of silence, shame, and concealed dread, prominent women began to share their breast cancer experiences in visible settings.[15] Breast cancer thus became a public matter during the 1970s when several notable pioneers pierced the quiet and the media seized on their stories. Shirley Temple Black, Happy Rockefeller, and Betty Ford, for example, went public about their surgeries, with the first and second ladies vigorously assuring publics of the success of their mastectomies. In 1974 a *Time* article praised Happy Rockefeller and Betty Ford for their "remarkable poise" in speaking out about their cancer experiences and mastectomies. "Their examples," the article argued, "should help thousands of others to overcome quite natural fears, and to learn the facts about a serious and little understood disease that once was discussed only in whispers."[16] Rockefeller's battle against cancer involved a second mastectomy for carcinoma in situ a few weeks after her first. In a move that reveals the lingering paternalism of the day, because of her "emotional state" Vice President Rockefeller and his wife's surgeons withheld the truth from her until the time of the surgery.[17] The paternalism entailed in this action preserved existing power structures, which placed doctors and husbands in charge. Barron Lerner has noted that during the 1950s and 1960s, most physicians of the day, in concert with patients' families, preferred not to disclose a cancer diagnosis.[18] Beyond protective paternalism, Vice President Rockefeller's decision reflects statistics of the day in a second way: according to Theresa Montini and Sheryl Ruzek, doctors performed forty-six thousand radical mastectomies in 1974, just slightly less than the sixty-five thousand performed in 1965.[19] Paternalism favored Halsted.

However, if the decisions of the first and second men on behalf of the first and second ladies preserved the status quo, other women formed a chorus of voices challenging the basis of physician paternalism. Indeed, a surge of breast cancer activism in the 1970s confronted and eventually transformed the doctor-knows-best model of patient care and nudged into place a restructured clinical relationship in which women could be active partners in their care. Women like fifty-year-old writer Babette Rosmond stared down physicians' professional authority when they refused to accept the Halsted radical mastectomy. "I, alone, am in charge of my body," Rosmond wrote in her 1972 book, *The Invisible Worm: A Woman's Right to Choose an Alternate to Radical Surgery.*[20] At this time, DC journalist Rose Kushner launched her campaign to involve women in their treatment, eventually going on the road with Bernard Fisher to promote more limited surgery. Meanwhile, Betty Rollin's *First, You Cry* and Audre Lorde's *The Cancer Journals* further challenged medical paternalism and expressed public grief about losing a breast.[21] Lorde, a noted black lesbian poet, bravely spoke to the indignities of her white prosthetic breast and the need to speak out. "My silences had not protected me. Your silence will not protect you," she wrote in an explicit call for active transformation of breast cancer politics.[22]

If Happy Rockefeller and Betty Ford—whose husbands chose treatment in concert with doctors—represented a blend of benevolent patriarchy marking the courage of women choosing to speak out, then Rose Kushner and Audre Lorde signified a new form of feminist breast cancer activism. Shaped by second-wave feminism and the women's health movement, Kushner's actions culminated in the 1986 founding of the National Alliance of Breast Cancer Organizations (NABCO), which serves as an information resource on the medical, psychological, and legal issues associated with breast cancer. While each of these women presented different models for challenging paternalism, their voices collectively contributed to a period of increasing public awareness, political organizing, and personal interest. Their efforts were critical to overturning silence about the topic and ushering in a new era of openness and conversation. As Susan Sherwin notes, "Breast cancer is now a familiar topic of news reports and documentaries, the target of numerous advertising campaigns, and the focus of significant fundraising efforts."[23]

In addition to pushing for increased education and awareness, women's efforts were crucial to gaining support for lumpectomy. In chapter 3 I chronicled Bernard Fisher's advocacy for lumpectomy; however, Fisher's success was bolstered by a tidal wave of activism in which women refused to consent to breast removal. Rose Kushner posed a question in 1975 that reflected the growing schism between women, their surgeons, and Halsted's radical mastectomy: "Why are most surgeons in the United States still doing the disabling Halsted radical when the modified radical is just as good?" she asked.[24] Kushner's activism reminds us that the gradual acceptance of lumpectomy reflected the achievements of not just Fisher and the NSABP but also of the women who fought for its adoption and the confirmation of its efficacy through grassroots support of critical research.

Indeed, grassroots organizing played a significant role in spreading awareness as self-help and local associations sprung up all over the nation. These groups reflected great ideological diversity and ranged from fairly conservative associations, such as the Susan Komen Foundation, to more radical green/environmental and feminist groups. Nonetheless, some research suggests that many groups tend to adopt conventional feminine gender roles and an apolitical guise. For instance, in her analysis of the politics of volunteers at the Susan Komen foundation, Amy Blackstone argued, "It is important to note that historically, women volunteers entered the world of politics and civic affairs at the same time that they remained the primary caretakers of their homes. In other words, while the first women volunteers may have been pioneers in a certain sense, they were not in others, for they did not challenge gender-based divisions of labor."[25] "Likewise," she continued, "heteronormative constructions of gender play out in the lives of individual Komen volunteers."[26] In a typical example: "Polly's daughter volunteers at the office during school breaks because her mom has had breast cancer and she wants to support her. Although Polly's husband also wishes to show his support for Polly, he does so by providing financial resources both directly to Komen and also to Polly so that she may work for Komen as a full-time volunteer."[27] Given Komen's popularity and the representative power of Polly's story, we might speculate that many women who participate in mainstream breast cancer organizing do so from traditional and conservative, rather than radical, political positions.[28] According to Blackstone, participation often stems more from the desire to volunteer for a worthy cause than to change underlying political structures that inhibit breast cancer research or to push for research into environmental carcinogens. "For Komen participants," she writes, "viewing what they do as simply fair, not political, is an essential aspect of their volunteer identities. This is linked to a traditional vision of gender in which politics is thought of as best left to men."[29] As breast cancer became more mainstream and less radicalized, it would be adopted as a cause by women from all walks of life, in partnership with a parade of corporate sponsors. In short, breast cancer became domesticated, at once mundane and ubiquitous though still scary, and subject to household, market, and corporate influences, as all of those pink ribbons and yogurt tops testify.

It is easy to see why breast cancer is an issue that most women—and their loved ones and corporate sponsors—can rally behind. After all, it is reputed to be the most common form of non-skin cancer found among women in the United States. The well-rehearsed statistics are these: Of the estimated 200,000 U.S. women and 1,000 men diagnosed with breast cancer each year, nearly 44,000 will die. Breast cancer is second only to lung cancer as the leading cause of cancer deaths in females in the United States. While a woman under age 39 has a 1 in 223 chance of developing breast cancer, the odds increase with age. By age 80, a woman has a 1 in 8 chance of developing breast cancer.[30] This probability is the one commonly cited in the mass media, but it does skew perceptions of the chance of developing the disease, since it is based on lifetime probability for a woman who lives more than eighty years, not the probability that a woman will develop cancer in a particular year. But more than the likelihood of being diagnosed with breast cancer, the disease strikes an erotically and culturally charged part of women's bodies. As Cherise Saywell notes, "Cultural anxieties about breast cancer are determined by the intersection of popular discourses of femininity and illness at the icon of the breast, and complicated by its status as diseased."[31] At once maternal, erotic, and feminine, breasts command significant attention. And the NSABP studies seemed to offer impetus to save them.

To put the complexities of Datagate into context and to explain the depth of frustration many women felt at the time, it is important to note that the controversy occurred amid a giant mobilizing effort of the National Breast Cancer Coalition, founded in 1991, which in the early 1990s had "taken Congress and the White House by storm."[32] Indeed, for months before the scandal broke, the NBCC had been working with Congress to raise awareness, funding, and stakeholder participation in breast cancer research initiatives. As Maren Klawiter has explained, "Almost overnight, it seemed, an astonishingly powerful breast cancer movement had converged on Washington," as NBCC "organized public marches, candlelight vigils, a demonstration on the front lawn of the White House, and rallies where 'breast cancer survivors'—a new collective identity and political actor—demanded more scientific research, medical progress, and public awareness of the disease."[33] The group was extremely effective at lobbying, securing more than $343 million dollars in research funding within its first two years.[34] Thus, when NBCC president Fran Visco spoke, she summoned the moral authority of a powerful and growing collection of voices. Moreover, NBCC's momentum helps to explain the frustration many women felt when they learned of Datagate, for its failures erupted at precisely the moment when the future for breast cancer research, treatment, and prevention seemed to be getting brighter.

I offer this abbreviated account of women's role in breast cancer advocacy not as an exhaustive picture of the gains over the course of the twentieth century; for that, readers can look to Barron Lerner's superb histories or to Ulrike Boehmer's *The Personal and the Political* and Maren Klawiter's *The Biopolitics of Breast Cancer*.[35] Instead, I want to bring readers who are unfamiliar with this history to the realization that women's participation in breast cancer advocacy emerged from a longer struggle that resulted in widespread, mainstream acceptance of increasing amounts of time, research, and money spent on women's health initiatives, particularly breast cancer. That the khaki uniforms of the Women's Field Army have been thoroughly replaced by ubiquitous pink ribbon paraphernalia, Races for the Cure, and Breast Cancer Awareness Month testifies to the success of efforts to cast breast cancer as a dominant political issue that men and women of all creeds—and corporations of all motives—stand behind. As Barbara Ehrenreich has wryly pointed out, "While AIDS goes begging and low-rent diseases like tuberculosis have no friends at all, breast cancer has been able to count on Revlon, Avon, Ford, Tiffany, Pier 1, Estee Lauder, Ralph Lauren, Lee Jeans, Saks Fifth Avenue, JC Penney, Boston Market, Wilson athletic gear," and the list surely grows.[36] Breast cancer has thus become "currently the most visible cancer in press coverage of health."[37] Yet, as Susan Sherwin has noted, "This coincidence of interests among medical, scientific, and commercial practitioners has led many feminists to wonder about how women's well-being fits into the agendas of these powerful interest groups."[38] This statement reveals the problematics of representation when powerful interests—corporate, biomedical, and advocacy groups of various stripes—are speaking for "women's" interests. Such collectivities can be powerful, they can achieve much, yet they can also push their broader agendas and interests at the same time. Perhaps nowhere is this vast collage of intersecting interests and motives more evident than in women's responses to NSABP Datagate and the rhetorical appeals and personae they forged in the process.

Before I turn to these responses, however, I want to make clear that even the framing of the issue in terms of women's health was contested. Although many women who spoke during Datagate did so first and foremost as women, others attempted to define the issues more broadly. Alisa Solomon has noted that "because it occurs in that iconic lump of flesh—both erotic and maternal—[breast cancer] brings the sexism in women's health issues to the surface."[39] Competing congressional testimony evinced a contest to characterize the situation as one of women's health versus scientific research in general. Harold Varmus, then director of the National Institutes of Health, tried to transition away from the testimony of the panel that spoke before him—the accounts of Jill Sigal, Cynthia Pearson, and Fran Visco—noting, "We've just experienced an emotionally trying discussion by three women who have all been affected by or are involved in the ramifications of the breast cancer studies that we've talked about. Ms. Sigal's testimony was particularly impassioned and moving." Retreating from "trying" emotion, Varmus wanted instead to "move into a more analytic mode to discuss the process by which the current events unfolded." Whether he intended to or not, he contrasted the emotionally feminine with the masculine analytical. Yet Varmus wanted to make sure that "although we are five men at this table responsible for some of the events . . . it is important to remember that we, too, have a deep, passionate involvement in these issues. In my own case, my mother and my grandmother died of breast cancer." Despite his familial connection to breast cancer, Varmus underscored that "we're not just talking about gender issues and breast cancer, we're talking about all of the research that's affected by NIH."[40] This framing was contested, however, as others repeatedly asserted that women's health was the matter at hand. Colorado representative Schroeder, for instance, following opening statements by John Dingell and Henry Waxman, thanked the subcommittee for "taking women's health seriously."[41] Thus, the congressional testimony over Datagate comprises a primary place where the quest to define breast cancer research as a women's issue or as a broader matter of scientific integrity becomes clear. However, in the overall vision, whether the issue was framed as one of women's health or not, participants often unwittingly scripted themselves out of active roles.

WOMEN'S RESPONSES TO DATAGATE

Responses to the controversy by individual women and the larger, collective advocacy groups that represented them were swift but varied. Making and answering telephone and hotline calls; sharing information and hosting support groups; defending or chastising their doctors and the medical establishment; and partnering with advocacy groups, other patients and the media afforded women and breast cancer organizations the chance to exert some degree of control over the situation. But most media accounts accentuated not the actions of women in response to the controversy but the uncertainty, insecurity, and anger women experienced in the wake of John Crewdson's *Chicago Tribune* article, which initially alerted the public to problems with NSABP data. The *New York Times* reported that "the revelation over the weekend that some data from a major breast cancer study were falsified has stirred an array of emotions among women who have undergone or are considering surgery that they hope will save their lives."[42] According to the March 25, 1994, issue of *Science,* Crewdson's exposé "touched off a wave of anxiety as women fretted over whether they had made the correct choice of treatment."[43] "Fretting," of course, is stereotypically the province of women, thus revealing the gendered nature of such coverage, which emphasized culturally conventional feminine affect. Would headlines report that men with testicular cancer "fretted" if their doctors falsified data?

Emotion and agency intertwined in ways that resonated long after Crewdson's.[44] Three years after the controversy, the narrative that women pulled their support from clinical trials was still routinely rehearsed. Barbara Weber, director of the breast cancer program at the University of Pennsylvania's Cancer Center recalled in the *Scientist* "a period of time during which women were confused about the [treatment] choices they had made or were worried about decisions they would have to make." "The announcement of the fraud," she said, "unquestionably had an effect on recruiting women into clinical trials."[45] Worried and wounded, fretting and anxious, yet capable of exercising agency by refusing to participate in medical trials, a stock construction of wounded and wary women emerged.

The degree of attention paid to the emotional responses of women to the news of data falsification in Datagate was a double-edged sword that risked stereotyping and infantilizing them at the same time that it brought into sharp relief the exquisite agony of uncertainty some of them felt regarding their condition. It is true that illness can diminish a sense of agency because of its existential threat, yet it can also endow a sense of agency by providing a larger sense of meaning, purpose, or direction. In the case of Datagate, the adjectives "terror," "agony," "fear," "anxiety," and "panic" pervaded the discourse. In most cases, newspapers featured women's emotions. "My Heart Stopped" began a section heading of the *New York Times* article "Flawed Cancer Study Haunts Many Women."[46] "My immediate reaction was panic," said Teresa Hanlon, a Pennsylvania schoolteacher who underwent a lumpectomy years earlier. Although Hanlon reported "calming down" and "honestly felt [she'd] made the [lumpectomy] decision five and a half years ago with a great deal of thought and a great deal of study," other women testified to preoccupation with whether the outcome of NSABP research would threaten their lives. "My heart stopped, literally," reported Anne Wheeler, who was then undergoing her final radiation treatment following lumpectomy. "This is a life decision I made based on data that said both worked equally well. I'm going through a lot. I don't want to question what I did and the choice I made."[47] "I was shocked," explained Columbia-Presbyterian breast surgeon Dr. Freya Schnabel. "When these things happen, it's better to air it out promptly and let everybody know about it right away."[48] While emotions triggered from Datagate ranged from apathy to anger, the focus on emotion, even as reassurances about the value of lumpectomy came pouring in, simultaneously revealed a sense of horror at the same time that it confirmed gender stereotypes of women as leading with their hearts over their heads. Even Dingell seized on the emotion trope to emphasize his broader agenda: "Women with breast cancer are widely reported to be 'devastated' and 'enraged,' with their confidence shaken both by the fraud and by the inexplicable delay in its revelation." Dingell reportedly shared this characterization with U.S. Department of Health and Human Services Secretary Donna Shalala in "an unusually blistering letter," thus showing how women's emotions could be marshaled in his campaign against big science.[49]

Reports of the degree of fallout conflicted, however, both while it was ongoing and years after the controversy had ended. "The fallout from the 1994 *Chicago Tribune* report of fraud was immediate, initially causing a slowdown in the rate at which women entered breast cancer clinical trials, cancer specialists note," maintained the 1997 *Scientist* essay "Observers Say Fisher Case Highlights Flaws in System."[50] "Many women questioned the integrity of researchers, trials, and their findings," and "wondered about lumpectomy as a treatment choice. Some physicians and others involved in clinical trials contend, however, that when people realized that the incident was an isolated one, public trust in science ultimately suffered little."[51] Nevertheless, accounts appearing as the controversy unfolded revealed divergent assessments, which can only have heightened the general confusion. *New York Times* science and health reporter Gina Kolata wrote on March 15, 1994, that "support organizations and groups like the American Cancer Society were flooded with calls from women, some worried that they had chosen the wrong treatment, others afraid that they now lacked reliable evidence on which to base a future decision."[52] "The number of calls to Y-ME has not been overwhelming, about 50 in the past 10 days," said a spokesperson to the *Chicago Tribune*, "but they have persisted. Other organizations around the country report moderate levels of concern, fueled mostly by the failure of the research study's organizers to make public data showing that their conclusions really are unaffected."[53] By contrast, journalist Robin Herman noted on April 19, 1994, that "the reaction of breast cancer patients to the lumpectomy scandal has been generally subdued. The NCI's office of cancer communications recorded no flood of anxious telephone calls. In fact, more consumer inquiries have poured in concerning the tamoxifen prevention trial and the changes in the guidelines for mammography for women under 50."[54] Thus, the rhetoric of reassurance of the NCI and the wave of concern from the ACS conflicts with varied accounts of how much this scandal affected patients.

However much public commentary was conflicted, women still sought advice from their personal physicians and still felt that oversight officials lacked respect in their responses to the controversy. "Despite all indications that the fraud has not altered the validity of the NSABP research, patients and doctors have been left to cope with the fallout," wrote Sheryl Stolberg in the *Los Angeles Times*. "Phones were active in the offices of breast surgeons and oncologists across the nation. 'I must have had 30 calls,' said Dr. Avrum Bluming, an Encino [California] oncologist."[55] Harmon Eyre, chief medical officer of the American Cancer Society, noted, "This is creating a substantial problem of trust and uncertainty. Women are challenging whether or not they had the right treatment, and doctors are concerned about how to respond."[56] Independent film producer and breast cancer patient Jane Alsobrook, who was serving on the board of a California breast cancer advocacy group, said, "It makes us angry that . . . [authorities] think it's not worth letting the general public know about unless somehow it leaks and creates a stir, and after the fact they say, 'Oh, yes, that did happen, but don't worry your little head about it.'"[57] Susan Tibbits, executive director of the National Association of Women's Health Professionals, echoed these remarks, noting that "what was missing here was a sense of responsibility to all of the women whose lives have been, are and will be affected by breast cancer." She cited a "lack of respect" on the part of "somebody" who "made a judgment that we are not going to share this information."[58]

Yet a sizable number of women wondered what was causing all the fuss. For example, Janet Perkins, a controller at an architectural firm in Atlanta, Georgia, noted, "I would have a little trouble understanding why there would be much concern about a nine-year-old study. There is a far longer history of this procedure in Europe. As has been the case with many treatments, the United States tends to lag behind. I think there has been sufficient data since then from actual practice that the results are very clear."[59] "'The present-day patient is pretty well educated, and they can handle the fact that some people are deceptive,'" Drummond Rennie asserted. "What they need are the facts to discuss with their doctor. And what the doctors need are the correct facts to talk with their patients.'"[60] In a representation that similarly afforded women more intellectual agency, the head of Johns Hopkins's Oncology Center noted, "There is something very impressive about the patients' reaction. They understand what goes into a clinical trial."[61] We thus discover a tension between a construction of women as sophisticated connoisseurs of the vagaries of clinical trials and as anxious women who are overly reliant on and supplicant to the testimony of the medical establishment, between women constituted as knowledgeable and resourceful and as helpless victims of the medical establishment.

Some women staffed phone lines. Marilyn Zwiers of Y-ME reported, "'The first call we got was the morning after the story broke . . . from a 51-year-old woman who had had a lumpectomy last October and was sure she had made the wrong decision.'" "That call was quickly followed by another from a recent lumpectomy patient," Zwiers told reporter John Crewdson, "a 67-year-old woman who also had heard the news and who Zwiers described as 'scared to death.'" The nine-year breast cancer survivor Zwiers's "litany" was that "there is no evidence that the fraud has affected the conventional wisdom that lumpectomy can be as safe as total mastectomy for women whose tumors are detected early." Another Y-ME administrator said, "'I think the concern is mainly, did I do the right thing? . . . Should I go back to my surgeon and have a mastectomy? We're telling them no, no one should run out now and have a mastectomy. We're telling them there are other studies and that most likely when this is over all the conclusions will still hold up.'"[62]

While some women's voices appeared in public by virtue of their having offered comments to newspaper reporters trying to meet deadlines, other women took more sustained public roles. Representing the face of both reassurance and technical sophistication, the renowned breast cancer physician Dr. Susan Love became a prominent voice in media stories about the case. As a leading international expert on breast cancer and a colleague of Dr. Fisher, Love faced competing allegiances to the research community, to her patients, and to Fisher. Karen Stabiner's *To Dance with the Devil: The New War on Breast Cancer* narrated Dr. Love's experience of being interviewed by ABC News at the UCLA Medical Center after Datagate. *To Dance with the Devil* presented Love as refusing to speak out against Fisher, because "she believed he was about to be crucified for what happened, and she refused to be part of it."[63] According to Stabiner, "While the cameraman set up his equipment, Love told the producer that everyone was overreacting. The lumpectomy study was still valid, and its findings were supported by other lumpectomy studies, so to say that the NSABP had duped a generation of women was a gross understatement. She could even understand Fisher's decision to hold back the information rather than needlessly frighten women."[64] Here, Love performed both a voice of reassurance of patients and a voice of a biomedical researcher. But while Love tried to reassure in an authoritative way, other women's efforts to provide information and context faced setbacks and reveal the dilemmas of trying to act in the face of uncertainty.

WOMEN FIGHT BACK: THE BATTLE AT BREAST CANCER ACTION OF MONTREAL

Sharon Batt's 1994 *Patient No More: The Politics of Breast Cancer* provides a rare glimpse into the behind-the-scenes struggles of patients and activists who tried to respond to the crisis. It also reveals the dilemmas of trying to serve diverse stakeholders, even when they are seemingly united under the banner of breast cancer. Batt recounts the efforts of the advocacy group Breast Cancer Action of Montreal (BCAM) in the days after the initial news reports of Poisson's deceit. She begins by describing her "astonishment" at reading a Canadian news report on March 13, 1994, after early morning phone calls from friends and reporters who had already seen the story. The Pittsburgh dateline attributed to John Crewdson, "City M.D. Tied to Research Fraud: U.S. Probe Casts Shadow on Key Breast Cancer Studies," prompted Batt's stunned realization that Poisson was practicing medicine a mile from her apartment.[65] Although she did not know Poisson personally, Batt soon heard from BCAM compatriots that Poisson had reached out to the group in the past; they described Poisson as "pleasant and genuine," and noted how rare it was for a doctor to contact them.[66] Before long, Batt herself gave voice to her concerns. "I am appalled," she testified to a Canadian reporter. "It's an incredible story. The ramifications are too big to even grasp."[67] These words appeared in the *Montreal Gazette* along with her observation that "That kind of abuse of power is really shocking and scary."[68]

BCAM mobilized quickly. The idea to host a meeting where past and present patients could air their concerns originated when one of Poisson's patients called Batt to ask if her group intended to "do something" in response to the news. Batt recounts that the woman said, "I feel isolated. The whole thing is eating at me. I'd like to meet with other patients, away from the hospital, and just talk about everything. Maybe together we can come up with a plan. I can't do it myself, but your group could sponsor a meeting."[69] BCAM did and formed an organizing committee, which included two patients from Saint-Luc Hospital. They booked a church hall and issued a press release. Telephone calls soon flooded BCAM members. As Batt recalls, "Some patients assumed the meeting was being called by the hospital. They asked if they needed to bring their files. Others stressed that they didn't want to see Poisson's reputation tarnished. He was a good doctor. Callers' interest was intense. So was their anxiety."[70] Even in patients' efforts to come to terms with what the tainted data meant for their battle against cancer, blaming and defending Poisson was prominent.

The politics of inclusion haunted the effort from the start. When Poisson's co-investigator and wife, Sandra Legault-Poisson, called to inquire about the meeting, Batt asked her not to attend, because "patients would be intimidated."[71] Concerned about the negative media coverage of her husband, Legault-Poisson showed up anyway with Poisson supporters, much to Batt's chagrin. Batt recalled asking Legault-Poisson to leave during a particularly tense moment when the press was, literally, banging the door down:

> "Dr. Legault . . . I asked you not to come."
> "I thought it would be best that I be here. I heard there would be re-porters."
> As we spoke, the TV journalist and his crew were banging at the door, explaining the sacred ritual of the set-up shot, trying to push through.[72]

Journalists, too, were not welcome. Finally, Legault-Poisson left the meeting, which offered her the opportunity to conduct media interviews outside the session, while BCAM members conducted their business behind closed doors. Just as Fisher's decision not to communicate the problems with Poisson's data to broader nontechnical audiences had consequences for his credibility, the desire of Batt and her colleagues to close the meeting so that it would serve patients also provided an opening for other rhetors to try to gain ownership over the issue. Canadian media framing of the meeting reflected the view of those excluded from the room, with *La Presse* noting the meeting had devolved into "squabbling," another stereotypically feminine trait.[73] This anecdote about BCAM's meeting thus reveals how both citizens and advocacy groups grappling with breast cancer decisions fell prey to some of the same media dilemmas as those facing Fisher and Poisson. The decision to confine communication had negative consequences in both cases.

Back inside the BCAM session, the fifty or so chairs arranged in a circle could not accommodate the eighty to one hundred people Batt estimates showed up. A woman named Denise opened the meeting by describing herself as "a patient at St. Luc, distraught by these revelations." BCAM, she said, was "a voice for women with breast cancer, an educational group that encouraged patients to be informed and in control of their situation."[74] Soon, the meeting that had been intended to provide solace turned rancorous. After one questioner who had had a lumpectomy wanted to know if it was the right treatment, the woman seated previously next to the now-absent Dr. Legault "cried, indignantly," that "a doctor who could have responded to your questions was asked to leave!"[75] Poisson supporters wanted to use the meeting to rehabilitate the reputation of their physician. Others wanted answers that nonc in the room could provide.

At one point a woman named Rose spoke out: "We all hope we had the right treatment," she said. "The problem is, our treatment is based on research. What we want for ourselves, and for our daughters, is accurate research, accurate information on which to base our decisions. We're not here to decide whether Dr. Poisson is a good doctor or not. We're here to talk about the consequences of falsifying research."[76] And so the conversation shifted to questions of blame, facticity, and future action. But it was exhausting. "All around," Batt noted, "faces showed the strain of agitation and fatigue."[77] In trying to provide a safe place for women to process their responses and find information and solace, BCAM, for all its good intentions, had unwittingly muddied the waters.

At the end of the meeting, Batt was confronted by the media when the TV journalist from Radio Canada noted that "People were upset that you couldn't answer their questions."[78] During BCAM's "post-mortem get-together" the group decided that "the evening was a disaster."[79] "Overnight," Batt testified, "our hard-won reputation as an articulate, coherent voice had acquired an ugly counterpoint—we were seen as raucous and divided."[80] This harrowing account of a public meeting gone awry illuminates the perils of agency and representation in such large-scale controversies, as efforts by women to do something for women after perceiving they had been harmed were denigrated for the same reasons as Fisher's silence about Poisson's data—for excluding key stakeholders. Trying to attend to the divergent needs of a diverse group of stakeholders at such a charged time quickly grew out of control. Thus, BCAM felt bound by the same set of media strictures as the doctors they criticized: others were trying to tell their story. Still, as other women weighed in on the controversy, the resultant personae provide opportunities for reflection about how our linguistic structures can curb or bolster efforts to participate in scientific processes and practices in cases where knowledge impinges on our daily life and welfare.

HUMAN GUINEA PIGS: WOMEN AS KNOWLEDGE CONSUMERS AND AS SUBJECTS OF SCIENCE

While it is not my aim to blame breast cancer advocates for the implications of their implicit characterizations, my analysis offers an account of how such characterization may unwittingly encourage or discourage particular lines of thinking and action. Moreover, I would be remiss in not pointing out that those who spoke during this controversy tended to represent the experiences of mostly white, middle- to upper-middle-class women with access to health insurance, doctors' offices, and the latest medical research and clinical trials, most of whom were diagnosed with early-stage breast cancers. Yet explicit attention to this subject position was muted in the controversy's discourse. Indeed, many politicians, consumer advocates, and breast cancer survivors who spoke in public about Datagate comprised rhetorically constituted characters enshrined in a political guise of non-politics. They represented the face of an abstracted, universal woman asking neither for explicitly feminist issues nor for radical changes in the system, but only for what was "fair." Representative Patricia Schroeder noted, "This is serious business, Mr. Chairman. We're talking about women's lives. We're talking about the integrity of the science behind treatment of a disease that will kill 46,000 women this year and afflict another 182,000. We're talking about research with a conscience."[81] "The bottom line in all of this," she argued, "is that quality of research translates into quality of treatment—and the trust people play in that treatment. And women have very little trust right now because their research has been compromised, resulting in many confusing signals."[82] Politically and rhetorically, this move to cast the issue in terms of research integrity was savvy in that it appealed to widespread notions about honesty and giving women their due, and thus muted racial and ethnic, class-based and political differences.

Schroeder's vision of research integrity built on a foundation of honesty and openness corresponded to one of the most dominant and arguably conservative characterizations to emerge during the controversy: that of women as knowledge consumers. Jill Lea Sigal's congressional testimony also embodied this construction. Like Schroeder, Sigal, too, cast the problem as one of accuracy and truth-telling. The job of scientists was to produce the truth and convey it to interested parties. "I mean, without this information being given to the doctors, the doctors can't advise people like myself adequately," Sigal explained under questioning.[83] Since Datagate compromised trust in NSABP research, then by extension, all data, all government research, became suspect: "I don't take their [NCI's] word for it," she testified. "I can't because my life is depending on this, as well as hundreds of thousands of other women. So, for them to tell me, oh, you're going to be OK, that doesn't mean anything to me today . . . Well, if it could happen in one study, maybe it could happen again."[84] Sigal's moving testimony emphasized "the fear that arises from facing one's own mortality at my age," which, she continued, "can at times be paralyzing. Now, as a result of this fraudulent study, and the apparent coverup by the National Cancer Institute and the University of Pittsburgh, my terror is exacerbated."[85] Sigal's youthfulness and emotional resonance conformed to wider cultural representations of women with breast cancer, since scholars have noted the "disproportionate representation of young women in media coverage."[86] Indeed, "breast cancer reporting is heavily preoccupied with youthful breasts, only occasionally focusing on the menopausal breasts most frequently affected."[87] Because of her emotional zeal and the cultural familiarity of her appeals to honesty, Sigal quickly became the face of women fighting for information; she epitomized the persona of the knowledge consumer.

The composite characterization of the knowledge consumer rested on a strict division between science and its stakeholders in which the former have an obligation to present timely information to the latter. This persona allowed women who were affected by breast cancer research to register outcry against scientific practices, but left them largely outside of technical decision making. The implied worldview of the knowledge consumer thus reinforced isolation between stakeholders and scientists by preserving for scientists the status of guardians of knowledge. Sigal's list of proposed correctives to the problems of Datagate vividly illustrated this separation. Her solutions included commissioning an independent analysis of NSABP data; ordering release of raw data with patient names redacted; extending Roger Poisson's eight-year debarment from federal funding to a lifetime; and changing the investigation, timeliness, and notification of scientific misconduct called "fraud." "Think about the agony of uncertainty that I and thousands of others are currently enduring," she admonished.[88] Yet none of these solutions asked for increased stakeholder participation in clinical trial design or research priorities; instead, they proposed the modest but understandable, commonsense, and certainly ethically defensible request for honesty and disclosure.

That the figure of the knowledge consumer pivoted on a sharp division between science and its stakeholders is evident across a swath of testimony. Representative Schroeder noted, "Consumers are not scientists. We know that. But we are not stupid, either. We don't want lies or sugar-coated results—just information, good information. We do not want to be patronized, especially in issues of life and death."[89] Dr. Trudy Bush at Johns Hopkins echoed this sentiment when she told the *New York Times,* "Women aren't stupid. We know mistakes can be made. We just want to be told the truth and make our own decisions."[90] Again and again, women represented the job of the scientist as to present the truth so that women could make their own decisions, a vision that comports with widespread social stereotypes about science as a product made by experts and consumed by lay people.

The touching story of Geri Barish, "who lost her mother to breast cancer," as rendered in the *New York Times,* also activated the knowledge consumer persona. "When she found a lump in her breast in June 1986," noted the *Times,* "the decision about what she should do weighed heavily on her."[91] Barish's story was saturated with tenets of the knowledge consumer, wherein truth-telling is the primary requirement for scientists involved in research that affects publics.

> In the end, Mrs. Barish, of Baldwin, L.I., said she based her choice on a study that said removing the tumor would be as effective as removing the entire breast. She had a lumpectomy.
>
> A year later, the cancer returned. And to learn now that the study she once believed in was based on flawed data has left her devastated.
>
> "I am furious," said Mrs. Barish, 50, who eventually had a mastectomy. "I'm wondering what else have they covered up? What else have they told us that is not true? I am very skeptical. And I'm very frightened."[92]

Barish's tale of skepticism and distrust illustrates how perceived breaches in trust can imperil decision making and create anxieties for patients who are trying to process the implications of technical information for their lives. Yet it also positioned women as the passive receivers of scientific knowledge, who could only register concern when something had gone awry.

Some representations of women during Datagate, including those made by and on behalf of women, further revealed the residue of a former victimhood construction. This vision tangled with more agentic images of women as capable knowledge producers and research collaborators. Representative Olympia Snowe noted, "The real terrifying impact of this research fiasco ultimately is on the victims, those women who have breast cancer, because they are going to be haunted by the notion as to whether or not they have made a correct decision; they are going to question the data, and the accuracy of the scientific information, and their doctor's recommendation. And who can blame them, Mr. Chairman?"[93] Depicting women as victims instead of relying on the survivor discourse resonated with commonsense assessments of the situation. In this view, because Fisher, Poisson, and oversight officials did not widely communicate Poisson's deception to the breast cancer community, they harmed patients and survivors; more pointedly, they victimized them. Women with breast cancer thus became double victims of both cancer and science. This framing provided an opening to cast women as victims of a hysterical media, since, according to the dictates of technical reason, there was no cause for alarm—the study's conclusions held even with Poisson's faulty data.

Although an alternate and more cynical read suggests that women were being used as pawns in a political battle to discipline big science, the victim view figured prominently in a discussion of Datagate that appeared in

Ladies' Home Journal in February 1995, less than a year after the scandal erupted. Andrea Rock's special report, "The Breast Cancer Experiment," rehashed the controversy, focusing on concerns about the tamoxifen breast cancer prevention trials that were also under NSABP purview and raising problems with breast cancer research more generally. The article concentrated on Washington, DC, attorney Laurel Neff, who on her thirty-third birthday, in 1982, submitted to a biopsy while her mother "lay dying from breast cancer."[94] Rock thus wove a pathos-heavy tale involving Neff's experience of being told she had a 25–33 percent chance of developing breast cancer, being presented with options ranging from doing nothing to double mastectomy, and deciding in 1992 to enroll in the NSABP tamoxifen trial. "Neff jumped at the chance to participate," Rock wrote, quoting the woman as saying, "It offered me the potential to escape my mother's fate and live to see my children grow up."[95] Rock characterized the process of joining the trial as arduous, requiring a yearlong series of exams and interviews. She signed consent forms listing the side effects of tamoxifen: "hot flashes, blood clots, eye problems, a slight risk of liver cancer and a slight risk of uterine cancer."[96] "Little did she know at the time," Rock dramatized, "but Neff was becoming involved in one of the largest and most controversial medical experiments ever involving women."[97] The "serious, even dangerous problems" of the trial included subjects who were "putting themselves at much higher risk of uterine cancer than the slight risk mentioned in the consent forms."[98] Rock's story dramatized the danger of women who participate in clinical trials as it rendered Neff and others like her both subjects of science and, hence, victims of its vagaries.

The victim characterization derived its power from its appeal to unknown harms to women because of their participation in the then reputationally challenged clinical trials. Even though other studies had demonstrated the value of lumpectomy, and even though officials had assured women that lumpectomy with radiation was still valid, this characterization persisted in its deep belief that women had been collectively wronged by science. It appealed to long-term familiar scars and traded on universal womanhood status borrowed from earlier rhetorical forms that privileged genteel womanhood. This construction in part explains the success of the breast cancer movement, which made breast cancer a mundane, consumerist, and mainstream issue, albeit one that benefited from corporate largesse. This characterization is in part based in a stark reality, but it also ceded women's subordinate status in clinical trials and thus constituted women as subjects of science. As Karen Stabiner noted, Fran Visco's response to the controversy "confirmed her worst fear—that researchers essentially operated in secret, as members of an exclusive society whose doors were closed to the women who made their studies possible."[99]

However, this construction of women as subjects of—that is, subjected to—science, used by the medical establishment but perpetually disrespected, was not unchallenged in public discourse. For example, Margaret Heuser of Montreal confronted the construction of women as victims and subjects of science when she tried to reposition research subjects as contributors to knowledge production. Heuser wrote to her hometown *Montreal Gazette* as a ten-year breast cancer survivor, tamoxifen taker, and past participant in an NSABP study: "At the time of my diagnosis," she observed, "I was offered a free choice between individual treatment or treatment within the research program headquartered in Pittsburgh (National Surgical Adjuvant Breast and Bowel Project, or NSABP). No pressure was brought to bear on me." Heuser argued that generalizing from Poisson's actions to all federally funded cancer research undermined the future of the entire research enterprise. "A wholesale attack on current cancer research has grown, more or less, out of one doctor's seriously faulty records," she offered, "and I get the distinct impression that the original misdemeanor has unfortunately afforded an opportunity for those disgruntled by present funding to try to advance their own causes—at the expense of the current research." Heuser's words represent a departure from much of the early discourse on Datagate in two senses. First, they chastised those who used Datagate as a means of airing past grievances about the cancer establishment. She particularly felt this tendency was occurring around tamoxifen, which she defended by noting that "attacks have been made on the use of tamoxifen because of a marginal chance of causing uterine cancer; this is a one-sided argument that disregards tamoxifen's proven usefulness in preventing further breast cancer, outweighing the slight risk." Second, Heuser minimized the extent of the breach of trust and located it squarely in Roger Poisson's "seriously faulty records." "I am eternally grateful," she concluded, "for the fine medical treatment I received, treatment that had evolved over a number of years of cancer research, so I hope that my contribution in joining the breast-cancer research program might help someone else."[100] With these words, she constituted her participation actively as someone whose clinical trial participation would help other women; no passive victim or disempowered consumer, Heuser was both an agent with options and a willing participant in knowledge production.

The tension between Heuser's construction of women as active participants in life-saving research and Rock's construction of them as unwitting victims betrays the residue of broader debates about the relationship between women and the biomedical establishment. As Maren Klawiter has demonstrated, a regime of medicalization in the early part of the twentieth century operated "through a *proliferation* of public and private discourses and practices, not a deficit, that breast cancer was constituted as a 'hidden' disease and women with breast cancer were constituted as its invisible victims." She explained that "inside the surgeon's office, the operating room, and the hospital setting, breast cancer patients were indeed surrounded by silence, lies, and dissembling."[101] Thus, the casting of women as victims who were thoroughly subject to and yet squarely outside of the scientific process resonated with broader cultural themes and the longer history of breast cancer research. A countervailing persona, however, posited a more agential image and afforded women a more prominent place at the table.

WOMEN AS KNOWLEDGE PARTNERS

Fran Visco's characterization of women and her emplacement of them alongside scientists epitomize what I am calling the knowledge partner persona, which coalesced from accounts of advocates who used Datagate to increase their appeals for greater participation in biomedical research. At the Dingell oversight hearing, Visco noted that while the testifiers were gathered because of the crisis over NSABP data, she felt "very strongly that we would do a larger disservice to women if we do not use this opportunity to ensure justice in the future. We must make it a matter of policy that consumers—breast cancer advocates—are involved at every stage of the research process . . . women must be a part of the research process if their best interests are to be fully assured."[102] According to Visco, her organization, the NBCC, released a statement in response to NSABP data falsification, noting, "A tenet of the National Breast Cancer Coalition policy agenda is that consumers—breast cancer advocates—belong at every level of the research process, from advisory boards to study sections at the agency level, to steering committees, data monitoring committees and IRBs [institutional review boards], at the institutional and study level."[103] Although her language still bore the residue of the term *consumer*, it differed from the implicit vision of Sigal's knowledge consumer in that it entailed increased participation across the board.

> In response to the public's outcry that information had been kept from it, a top official of NCI was quoted as saying that if a year or two ago he had "intuited" women's concerns to the NCI/NSABP behavior, NCI would have acted differently. There is a fundamental defi-

ciency in a system where a public servant believes he must intuit how the public may react to decisions made by his agency. Had a consumer advocate—a woman with breast cancer—been part of the process, the public's peace of mind and women's lives would not have been left to the uncertainties of an individual's intuitive abilities. The self-imposed separation between the public agencies and the citizenry they serve is unacceptable.[104]

Visco thus requested a reframing of the role of publics in scientific life, which entailed greater incorporation of public inputs.

Cynthia Pearson's testimony on behalf of the National Women's Health Network similarly created a composite vision of the knowledge consumer and the knowledge partner. At the time, NWHN represented four hundred local women's health groups and boasted a membership of more than seventeen thousand.[105] They advocated for both improved health policies for women and better information. Resonating with the demands of the knowledge consumer, Pearson noted that NWHN's "biggest complaint" was "the delay of over a year in announcing to the public that falsified data were submitted to the NSABP."[106] She lambasted Fisher for his silence in not telling the women of America about problems with NSABP data and with the Breast Cancer Prevention Trial, calling his "disregard for the public's right to know . . . outrageous."[107] She echoed Visco's call for more participation at the same time she called for Congress to ensure a scientific review of NSABP research, thus blending the normative visions of both personae.

The knowledge partner shares in common with the knowledge consumer the passionate longing for purity, the desire for science to have gotten it right. The knowledge partner also demands disclosure of relevant information. However, Pearson transcended information sharing to ask for a "place at the table" and to explicitly call for bridges between science and publics. For instance, Fran Visco recognized that "Dr. Fisher was a visionary in the field of breast cancer. And that his leadership in this area was in part responsible for the advances that have been made." Nonetheless, Visco also noted that "when we concentrate too much power in too few people, we do a disservice to the public. I have seen what the individual, professional, and institutional ego can do: those in power get to a point where they become insulated from the public and from the patients they serve."[108] To counter such insulation, for Visco and others like her, participation in biomedical research processes by those affected by the research was imperative. Visco was emphatic about this point, both in her testimony and elsewhere. "With a diagnosis of breast cancer," she explained, "we find ourselves in a world over which we have little control. We have to learn a new scientific language. And we do. We have to understand new concepts. And we do. And we are asked to turn ourselves over unthinking, unquestioning to the scientific and medical communities. We do not. Not any longer.... We women with breast cancer, consumer advocates belong at the table."[109] Visco's testimony highlighted the dilemmas of stakeholder exclusion from the planning, execution, and communication of biomedical research. Declaiming the outsider status of those who have the biggest stake in the outcomes of federally funded research, she revealed the deleterious effects that women's lack of participation in breast cancer research could have on their lives and well-being.

The contrasts between women as knowledge consumers, as subjects of science, and as knowledge partners disclose an implicit struggle over women's identity and participation in breast cancer research: Were women duped by reticent scientists hesitant to expose the wrinkles in their data, were they rendered little more than the status of lab rats, were they left out of the communication loop, or were they capable participants who can weigh in on matters scientific? Viewed together, the knowledge consumer and the subject of science testify to the dominance of consumer models of health care, which relegated women outside of the scientific process. This observation underscores why it is crucial that rhetorical critics attend to the underlying vision of science conveyed in these otherwise seemingly mundane characterizations rather than uncritically accepting them as natural or inevitable. One way of achieving this aim is to deconstruct the implied relationships between science and its stakeholders, between biomedical research and researchers and the users and beneficiaries of that research. By exposing these implied relationships, we can better conceive of places for rhetorical invention and action, for these characterizations reflect the outcomes of a collective sense-making process in which representations of women influenced opportunities for their participation in biomedical research and reframed the relationship between science and stakeholders on a practical level. Thus, this case allows us to witness how rhetorical choices impinge upon issues of practice and policy. If the dominant rhetoric is one asking for truth-telling, then policy solutions aimed toward ferreting out transgressors who pollute science more readily appear in our linguistic and practical horizon. Viewed in this light, it is therefore not surprising that federal regulations requiring more meaningful participation of stakeholders in research were not forthcoming. Although the NSABP proposed having a community representative in their response to the controversy and did involve women in later research planning, some commentators called these mere public relations exercises. Fixes that involved audits and more monitoring were the predictable results at higher levels, preserving the schism between scientists and many of their stakeholders and engendering few, if any, structural changes between them.

Visions of women and their roles in breast cancer research further became a rhetorical vehicle for other stakeholders to the scientific process. The discourse of John Dingell, a powerful advocate known for bringing high-profile scientists to their knees, stressed the harms to women during the first of his two hearings devoted to "Fraud in Breast Cancer Research." On April 13, Dingell noted, "Because of the comments of Ms. Sigal, Ms. Visco, and Ms. Pearson, we're seeing [the issue] now from a more personal standpoint, from the hurt, the danger, the peril, the trauma that it occasions to citizens who, interestingly enough, are taxpayers who support these programs, who are entitled to openness and truth, who are entitled to honorable and proper behavior by investigators, and proper discipline within the scientific community and within the government itself."[110] Stirring up a dense cauldron of fear and emotion, Dingell thus positioned himself as guardian and watchdog of big science, as a protector of women, whom he characterized as traumatized by Datagate; but his self-casting, as we shall see, was not unblemished.

THE POLITICS OF BREAST CANCER AS BIG SCIENCE: JOHN DINGELL, "POLITICAL PROTECTOR" AND "DARK KNIGHT" OF SCIENCE

That breast cancer is a thoroughly political affair is by now a well-rehearsed point. What bears mention, however, is how the Datagate controversy intersected with a major initiative to discipline big science, spearheaded by Congressman John Dingell. During the late 1980s and early 1990s, the Michigan representative launched a series of high-profile efforts to stamp out abuses in big science. These hearings prompted a parade of big-name scientists testifying before the federal government. Scores of scientists faced the challenge of defending their actions and character before Dingell and wider mixed audiences, who may or may not have understood or cared about the scientific issues at hand. For example, Nobel Prize–winning biologist and Rockefeller University president David Baltimore, Stanford president Donald Kennedy, and former National Institutes of Health director Bernadine Healy were three scientists whose encounters with Dingell diminished their professional standing and raised doubts about their integrity. None of these hearings went particularly well for the scientists involved. As Wade Roush put it in 1992, "All three crossed Dingell in hearings conducted by his subcommittee—

and all three are still licking their wounds."[111] These three have since been cleared of wrongdoing, yet their experiences as scientists who were called to explain their actions in public serve as the backdrop to Datagate, because almost as soon as news reached the public following the *Chicago Tribune*'s initial article on the falsification, a furor followed, and Representative Dingell wasted little time in calling congressional subcommittee meetings to expose the perils of big science.

Dingell's tone and investigative zeal, both honed from his days as a prosecutor, were roundly dreaded in the scientific community. Dr. Bernadine Healy, who had previously faced Dingell's scrutiny, reported that "she was advised before the hearing to walk in on her knees 'so they can't kick you in the shins.'" She recalled replying, "But then they'll take my head off."[112] Other scientists echoed Healy's trepidation. As one unnamed researcher told *Science* magazine in 1991, "People are absolutely terrified of this Dingell business. They're afraid to make a mistake."[113] "But for the grace of God it could happen to any of us" said one NCI researcher with eighteen years of experience.[114] In the view of many members of the scientific community, Dingell was enacting the role of inquisitor, yet some members of the general citizenry lauded him as a champion of patients' rights.

The Dingell subcommittee hearings were motivated, at least according to explicitly stated reasons, by Dingell's belief that the scientific community had "been treated as a sacred cow for far too long" and needed to become more accountable to the public.[115] Indeed, Dingell's efforts to bring big science to task through well-publicized hearings were dubbed by critics as the "Dingellization" of science.[116] "Dingell thinks big-time scientists are given too much slack, that no one calls them into account, that big scientists are arrogant and insensitive," said one health official in 1994.[117] To date, there have been at least two book-length treatments of high-profile science controversies that landed before Dingell's hearings. Both illuminate Dingell's investigative prowess. The first, historian Daniel J. Kevles's *The Baltimore Case*, which examines Dingell's pursuit of David Baltimore, reveals Dingell's enlistment of secret service agents to collect evidence against key scientists in the case. The second, reporter John Crewdson's *Science Fictions*, examines the high-profile battle over credit for discovery of HIV between Robert Gallo and France's Luc Montaigner.[118] My interest here is not to rehearse previous arguments about the benefits and harms of Dingell's self-proclaimed crusader status. Rather, I want to examine the dilemmas inherent in the political personae of public protector and the problems of ventilating science in public. Wade Roush christened Dingell a "Dark Knight of Science" for his "crusade" against misconduct in big science. This framing of his persona is an apt one, I think, in that Dingell simultaneously tried to defend publics from the perils of science unchecked while at the same time alarming the citizenry and calling to task scientists who were eventually exonerated.[119]

While much of the scholarly attention to Dingell's hearings has focused on the cases of Baltimore and Gallo, several less-high-profile cases also dampened lives and upended careers. In 1991 Dingell alleged in a public hearing that Cleveland's Rameshwar Sharma, a biochemist, had committed misconduct even though Sharma had been exonerated by the Office of Scientific Integrity the year before. Dingell's aides met with OSI officials to reconsider the case after Sharma had already been officially cleared by their own committee. According to Jock Friedly, "it took a panel of federal judges to conclusively vindicate Sharma," who, after the Dingell fiasco, lost his job, could not find academic employment, wracked up $250,000 in legal expenses, and considered ending his life. Regrettably, "the panel found that the original charges stemmed from a single, obvious and insignificant, typographical error."[120] Though vindicated, Sharma noted in 1997 that "to this date, I have not received a letter of apology" from Dingell, and "he has hurt me." Dingell "has never met me," Sharma said. "He has never asked my side of the story. He's a congressman and he's supposed to uphold the Constitution of the United States of America. Why is he hurting an innocent person?"[121]

If Dingell engendered fear and loathing from scientists, the second-generation career politician earned praise from other audiences for many of his investigative efforts. In fact, just months after the Fisher hearings in 1994, Dingell and his wife, Debbie, received the Betty Ford Award from the Susan G. Komen Breast Cancer Foundation for their work on breast cancer health issues at an annual awards luncheon in Dallas, Texas.[122] His concern for women's health during Datagate could only have better positioned him for this award. Meanwhile, outside of the scientific arena, Dingell enjoyed plaudits for ferreting out waste and fraud. It was widely reputed to have been Dingell's committee that exposed the Pentagon's $640 toilet seat in a move that spurred the reverse of exorbitant defense costs in the 1980s. Dingell also toppled Ronald Reagan's top White House aide, Michael Deaver, and routed out corruption in the generic drug industry, thus leading to drug policy reform. Despite praise from some audiences, Jock Friedly noted that these same actions could be interpreted as opportunism and that they have even been criticized for having caused additional harm. "Pentagon procurement officials," Friedly explained, "still insist that the $640 toilet seat was neither a 'seat,' nor, despite legend, the result of a Dingell probe."[123] Moreover, "numerous industry watchers and government officials say that Dingell's charges against drug and medical device manufacturers, though successful in rooting out widespread fraud, directly resulted in a slow-down in approvals of life-saving products."[124] Dingell's pursuit of fraud and corruption spanned the fourteen years up to 1994, when the Republican's Contract with America spurred reorganization of the House, meaning Dingell no longer held a chairmanship of the House Committee on Energy and Oversight.[125]

During the Datagate hearings, part of Dingell's rhetorical strategy was to adopt a no-nonsense, commonsense, "simple folks" style, as exemplified in the following exchange with the NCI's Harold Varmus during the NSABP hearings:

> Mr. Dingell: Now, let's look at this situation. Here we've got the University of Pittsburgh. Now, here the University of Pittsburgh solicited a million dollars from Zeneca for the endowment of a chair. They wound up getting $600,000. This is while a test of this particular pharmaceutical [tamoxifen] is going on. Does that seem quite cricket? Dr. Varmus, do you want to comment?
>
> Mr. Varmus: I personally have concern about engaging in that kind of relationship.
>
> Mr. Dingell: I wonder. Does it pass the Aunt Minnie Sniff Test?
>
> Mr. Varmus: What test? I'm sorry.
>
> Mr. Dingell: If Aunt Minnie were to sniff this, what would she say?
>
> Mr. Varmus: Can you explain the test to me, sir?
>
> Mr. Dingell: Well, Aunt Minnie is somebody we use around here because she has a sensitive nose. What we're trying to figure out is would she like the smell of this or not.
>
> Mr. Varmus: Probably not.[126]

In contrast to the elite technical language, qualified arguments, and obfuscations of scientific discourse, folksy flourishes such as the "Aunt Minnie Sniff Test" suggested that the scientist's knowledge in a specialized area could be countered by the practical common sense of an everyday person like "Aunt Minnie." Although Dingell framed himself, his Aunt Minnie, and his subcommittee as neutral watchdogs of abuses in taxpayer-funded research, as of 1997 all of the big-name scientists he took to task were ultimately vindicated—yet he gained political capital from his hearings.[127]

Dingell called this first Datagate hearing to order by framing the issue in stark terms, noting, "Today the subcommittee will examine a number of important issues associated with serious falsification and fabrication of data in some of the Nation's most important clinical trials on the treatment and prevention of breast cancer, the National Surgical Adjuvant Breast and Bowel Project, NSABP, led by Dr. Bernard Fisher of the University of Pittsburgh." He continued by framing the issue in terms of public trust: "A particular focus of this hearing is the Federal Government's response to these problems. This case has major implications for thousands of patients who have participated in NSABP studies for decades, for the American taxpayers who have funded NSABP studies in amounts in excess of $100 million, and for maintaining public trust in the integrity of science." With this pronouncement, Dingell highlighted the potential significance of misconduct in the NSABP research. Although the argument that the B-06 lumpectomy trial's conclusions were unchanged by Poisson's actions had been well circulated by this time, this fact was not high on Dingell's list of announcements. Instead, he chose to link the controversy to what he felt, "regrettably," was "only the latest in a series of cases the subcommittee has felt it necessary to examine." After reminding listeners that the subcommittee's "involvement in examining, investigating, and monitoring the handling of scientific cases dates back to 1988 when the subcommittee held its first hearing on the issue," he argued that many members of the scientific community had resisted outside scrutiny. "But as we see today," he observed, "scientific misconduct is a very real problem that requires an intensive and aggressive response by the scientific community itself and by the Federal Government." The case at hand, he argued, "is a vivid reminder of how poor the response of the scientific community can be and how serious consequences may be when the scientific community and the Federal Government fall down on the job."[128] Note that Dingell characterized this case as a "vivid reminder" of the issue that had become one of his overarching political pet projects, meaning that the Datagate controversy, with its breast cancer patients and a notoriously imperious scientist—afforded him a prime rhetorical exigence for his larger campaign to chastise big science.

It is hard not to regard Dingell's motivations as vexed when he summoned Fisher, an icon of breast cancer research, to Washington, particularly since Dingell may have been smarting from the lack of a formal finding of research misconduct in his previous project, the infamous "Baltimore affair." Dingell's participation in these scandals reveals the problematic of federally funded science. When science becomes a public good, it is subject to oversight by those whose motives may stem from altruism but may likely emanate from a complex stew of competing drives and political agendas. Science then becomes subject to the arguments of nontechnical reasoners in nontechnical forums. For a politician, calling out fraud in breast cancer, the dreaded darling of corporate and public interest, could certainly curry political support. Yet Dingell's no-nonsense renegade-for-truth persona orchestrated the public disciplining of many scientists in a way that both helped and harmed science and both helped and harmed citizens. To the extent that it signaled a clarion call for science to consider its public effects it was potentially useful, but to the extent that it unnecessarily humiliated innocent scientists and alarmed patients and the general citizenry it cultivated a landscape of fear, ignorance posing as knowledge, and anger. In short, it painfully exposed the chasm between science and publics, and in Datagate women with breast cancer were caught in the middle.

WOMEN, RHETORIC, AND AGENCY IN DATAGATE

Gains made by the women's health movement during the 1970s and 1980s meant that women entered clinical trials in increasing numbers while entertaining reasonable hopes that their care providers would treat them as able partners in their treatment plans. Datagate exposed rifts in this vision, revealing, in the worst case, a lingering, arrogant paternalism and, in the best case, a genuine—if misguided—desire not to unduly worry patients with unnecessary technical details that did not affect the general contour and outcomes of research. In a more charitable reading of Datagate, however, scientific administrators decided disclosure would have produced more alarm than enlightenment, since there were no changes to the lumpectomy data when Poisson's discrepant figures were removed. Yet many women vigorously protested this view, airing their hopes for enhanced communication, transparency, respect, and inclusion, and in the process they constructed visions of their ideal relationships to science and scientists.

In 2001, a mere seven years after Visco and Sigal spoke to Congress about Datagate, legal scholar and bioethicist Rebecca Dresser opined that "today, more than ever, biomedical research is a public affair." "A new breed of patient advocate," she noted, "sits at the table with scientists and policymakers, setting research agendas, planning studies, and considering how study results should affect clinical practice."[129] Dresser's new breed of advocate—present but, I argue, containing much untapped potential—had been a long time in coming. Indeed, women's efforts to participate more meaningfully in breast cancer research, to take but one example, resulted from a hard-won struggle that spanned the course of the twentieth century. Yet in 1994 such efforts seemed to have suffered a stunning setback when Sigal's and Visco's testimonies, along with those from a panel of other witnesses, exposed the painful consequences of women's exclusion from fundamental aspects of breast cancer research.

Efforts to speak for and represent the women impacted by NSABP research and the composite characterizations that resulted present implicit visions of what Sonja Foss, William Waters, and Bernard Armada term "agentic orientation"—that is, "a pattern of interaction that predisposes an individual to a particular enactment of agency."[130] Agency has been subject to fierce debates in communication studies concerning the extent to which individuals are origins of discourse and have the ability to influence the world around them.[131] Poststructural critiques of agency deny the subject as seat of origin of speech and question whether subjects "speak" discourse or whether discourses speak through subjects.[132] Regardless of one's philosophical stance on this matter, those who spoke out during Datagate did so with the expectation that their words mattered. In this way, the composite personae and collective identity of the women implicated by Datagate reveal underlying assumptions about the power of women to effect change in scientific research that materially affects their lives. For Foss and colleagues, "an agentic orientation generates an outcome tied to the choices made concerning structure and act. If agency is action that influences or exerts some degree of control, an agentic orientation must attend to the outcomes generated by particular enactments of agency."[133] And thus the composite characterizations of women as knowledge consumers, partners, or subjects of science during Datagate positions women as outside, inside, or victims of scientific research and practice. What shines through in the words of Visco and Pearson is not just the attention to the issues of women's health advocacy but also the demand for inclusion in all aspects of the research process; their words evidence a politics of reclamation and collaboration that stands in sharp contrast to the consumer persona. The tension between the knowledge consumer and the knowledge partner cuts across many fields of biomedical and scientific research; there are no easy ways of reconciling these two roles. Both accurate information and active participation in research are needed. The perennial question regarding such opposing characterizations, of course, is who benefits from perpetuating the characterizations of knowledge consumer, partner, or subject of science?

Albeit perhaps unwittingly, the knowledge consumer persona, despite its explicit critique of scientific practice, propped up the status quo and contributed to a continued separation between science and its stakeholders. It thus served biomedicine as an institution and the corporations and government agencies that fund it by masking the underlying political relationships and coinciding interests between them. This characterization ultimately buys into what Zillah Eisenstein has called a "cancer establishment," the confluence of the ACS, NCI, the FDA, and the EPA, which "articulate a cohesively authoritative breast cancer narrative" that "features cure over prevention, patentable and/or synthetic chemicals over natural and holistic methods."[134] The knowledge partner persona, by contrast, challenges the underlying separation between science and stakeholders calling for increased participation of women in research processes that affect them. The dangers inherent in such participation include the potential for cooptation by biomedical institutions, but the benefits include being able to secure a place at the table and bring important political issues to the surface. "An agentic orientation," Foss and friends tell us, "first takes into account structural or material conditions because every act is an interpretation of a set of conditions. Agency is 'always agency toward something,' and that something is the perceived structure."[135] And thus we see the underlying structures of science largely unchallenged in many mainstream responses to the controversy.

Although Datagate was hardly the first time women had raised concerns about the conduct or direction of federally funded breast cancer research, the scandal offered the opportunity for a sustained and publicized ventilation of grievances, and in the process implicit visions of the relationships between women, politics, and science were forged.[136] This chapter discerned the composite characterizations of women and their advocates who spoke out—or who were spoken about—concerning breaches in breast cancer clinical trials in the wake of Datagate. Although their voices do not coalesce into neatly recognizable characters in the same way as those of Poisson and Fisher in chapters 2 and 3, they instead attest to the complexity and multiplicity of subject positions and relationships to science. The journalistic representations of women's responses—anxious and existentially panicked, angered at nondisclosure, confused about treatment options, seeking to reassure others, and showing subdued concern—undoubtedly reflected the divergent responses of real women as they grappled with the meaning of the Datagate case for individual lives. Nonetheless, amplified by the mass media they become symbolic condensations, portraying an angered and anxious collective that afforded women—representing their individual breast cancer experiences, their family's breast cancer experiences, large advocacy coalitions, and breast cancer movements—the chance to air their views in a highly publicized series of congressional hearings. Nonetheless, women and others who participated in the critique of their medical institutions did align with several central visions: they appealed to honesty and truth-telling as knowledge consumers, they appealed to the right to participate in scientific research design, and they appealed to victimhood status. The political implications of these positions bear scrutiny.

Barbara Ehrenreich has noted that "breast cancer would hardly be the darling of corporate America if its complexion changed from pink to green."[137] Ehrenreich's comments strike at the core of one of the fundamental rhetorical constraints of women who spoke out against Datagate—their need to appear "reasonable," not too angry, not too vulnerable, not too feminist, and altogether mainstream. Despite, or perhaps because of, the success in making breast cancer a mainstream political issue, many made the case for participation in breast cancer research from apolitical guises. Cindy Pearson, former director of the National Women's Health Network, noted that "breast cancer provides a way of doing something for women, without being a feminist."[138] This finding resonates with research conducted by Amy Blackstone that women in some breast cancer advocacy groups actively maintain an apolitical guise.[139] Regardless of whether this view held in Datagate, the controversy provided an opportune moment to assert the need for broader reforms in women's health care. Striking a reasonable, mainstream core with the knowledge consumer and subject of science characterizations comported with dominant cultural values but preserved the division between scientists and a large number of stakeholders.

In sum, Datagate commanded attention in part because its spectacle of humbled scientists, angry politicians, and fearful patients provided a riveting opportunity for processing collective longings and anxieties about science and its position in our social world; audiences looked on with a mix of queasy fascination and existential dread. On the one hand, the controversy could be interpreted as a moment where those whose lives mattered the most—women with breast cancer—were systematically disrespected and ignored. On the other hand, it could be read as a triumph where women affected by breast cancer seized the moment to register their concerns and challenge the status quo. Neither of these visions adequately reflects the complexity of responses to Datagate or its multiple and contested meanings. Instead, Datagate reveals a simmering stew of motives, actions, constraints, and possibilities for science and its stakeholders and publics. Entanglements of power and hierarchy, authority and expertise, and knowledge and misinformation vexed this controversy from the outset, and they continue to do so.

If we look for a moment beyond the confines of the Datagate controversy, women's struggles in breast cancer advocacy still confront several obstacles. These include the persistence of mastectomy, the lack of investigation of environmental causes of cancer, and the remaining gap between science and the citizenry. First, in terms of mastectomy, as late as 2002, Monica Morrow noted in the *New England Journal of Medicine* that "despite a large body of mature scientific data from randomized trials, which is unequaled in the literature on the local treatment of cancer, many women today are not offered the option of breast conserving therapy."[140] This data suggests the need for more political action to ensure that all women, especially poor women, nonurban women, and women of color, are afforded access to breast conserving therapies. Second, while many activists have tried to "greenwash" the "pinkwash" of rhetoric that places responsibility on individual women and looks to personal rather than environmental causes, the dominant rhetoric does not readily accommodate environmental links that many argue have been suppressed.[141] Third, immediately after Datagate, the NSABP drafted a report asking for a consumer advocate to advise the NSABP on their studies. And although women are more routinely participating in lay and citizen advisory capacities in publicly funded science, private science lags behind. In their study of patients participating in research decisions in the Netherlands between 2000 and 2003, J. Francisca Caron-Flinterman and her coauthors found that "decision-making on biomedical research agendas, on individual levels, as well as on institutional and national levels, is mainly the territory of experts." Caron-Flinterman and her colleagues maintain that their findings apply to other nations and sites, thereby suggesting a continued need to integrate stakeholders more snugly into the fabric of scientific processes that affect their lives, to secure Visco's vision, that opened this chapter, of a place at the table.[142] Given this call, chapter 5 will consider reconfigurations of the relationship between science and those whose lives depend on it.

5

Recharacterizing Science and Public Life

Trust, Dialogue, and Citizen Engagement

As I conclude this book, headlines continue to deliver sensational tales of scientists cheating their way to fame and fortune. "Fraud Rocks Anesthesiology Community," reported *Anesthesiology News* in March 2009, dramatizing the story of falling star and pain management pioneer Dr. Scott S. Reuben, who stands accused of fabricating data in twenty-one studies published in leading anesthesiology journals since 1996.[1] Detailing "what may be among the longest-running and widest-ranging cases of academic fraud," the *New York Times* revealed that officials at Baystate Medical Center in Springfield, Massachusetts, have determined that the influential anesthesiologist committed "massive" research misconduct in studies that have direct implications for postoperative pain management.[2] Media coverage and medical journal articles suggest that Rueben is not alone: In 2001 international papers narrativized the deception of South African oncologist Werner Bezwoda, whose fabricated clinical trial data allegedly demonstrated the efficacy of high-dose chemotherapy with bone marrow transplant for advanced breast cancer.[3] In 2003 the *New York Times* reported that University of North Carolina researcher Dr. Steven A. Leadon resigned after allegations that he faked data in breast cancer research on tumor suppression, while in 2008 news outlets reported that Big Pharma had hidden less than glowing results from its antidepressant studies.[4] In short, the makers of Prozac and Paxil were not disclosing trial results showing that their products provided only modest gains over a placebo in fighting depression.

Amid these disturbing reports appeared the shocking story of the iconic South Korean stem cell researcher Dr. Hwang Woo-suk, whose "spectacular fraud" shook the international scientific community in 2005. Prior to the news that he fabricated data, the "charismatic" Dr. Hwang had captured public interest a year earlier when his coauthored *Science* articles announced stunning breakthroughs in embryonic stem cell research.[5] "The papers transformed Dr. Hwang into a national hero," explained one writer, "a handsome 53-year-old scientist who had risen from humble origins to lead South Korea to places it and the rest of the world had not seen. Web sites went up in his honor, women volunteered to donate eggs, Korean Air volunteered to fly him anywhere free."[6] The national mood turned from adulation to humiliation, however, when news that Dr. Hwang had made up data, which was used in his now apparently false claims to have cloned embryonic stem cells, circulated among front-page headlines of the same international newspapers that had trumpeted his success. As the South Korean government rushed to remove his accomplishments from science textbooks and halt production of a line of Hwang commemorative stamps, Hwang offered a tearful apology and explained the pressures he faced: "I was crazy with work . . . I could see nothing in front of me. I only saw one thing and that is how this country called the Republic of Korea could stand straight in the center of the world."[7]

Like Poisson's misguided data falsifications, Reuben, Bezwoda, Leadon, and Hwang's deceptions signal the particularly high stakes of health research where patients' lives are tightly yoked to scientific integrity.[8] In Poisson's case, news of data falsification compromised trust in federally funded breast cancer research. In Reuben's, Bezwoda's, and Leadon's cases, what experts believed to be true turned out to have been built on a foundation of lies. In Hwang's case, South Korea's scientific reputation plummeted when its iconic scientist tumbled from grace. These incidents recall Walter Ong's observation that science hinges on trust. As Ong reminds us, "Science itself cannot live save in a network of belief." "Even in the most 'objective' of fields," he explained, "the word of persons is more pervasive than factual observation."[9] Believing in the words of other scientists is a necessary condition for the contemporary clinic, laboratory, newspaper, and scientific journal office. Yet trust and truth are tangled in complexity, and when they are compromised or challenged, character becomes a mechanism for assessing the integrity of scientific claims.

In this book I have sought to rehabilitate trust and character as significant features of publicly debated scientific research. The idea that character makes a difference to the outcomes, meanings, and receptions of science may seem outmoded in our fragmented, postmodern, globalized world, where cynicism reigns and the very idea of a subject—much less one with an old-fashioned virtue like character—has been thoroughly deconstructed.[10] Yet nothing could be further from the truth. Precisely because the science that underwrites everything from public policy to medical treatment is increasingly conducted by agglomerated but far-flung strangers, the character of those who produce it has arguably never been more important. As I was finishing this book, the science historian Steven Shapin made a similar point in *The Scientific Life: A Modern History of a Late Modern Vocation*: "The closer you get to the heart of technoscience, and the closer you get to the scenes in which technoscientific futures are made," he wrote, "the greater is the acknowledged role of the personal, the familiar, and even the charismatic."[11] Shapin tracked changing perceptions of what it meant to be a scientist from the early modern envisioning of scientists as "priests of nature" through the early mid-twentieth-century idea of their "moral ordinariness," which posited the absence of personal influences on science and promoted the desirability of scientists' moral equivalence. Shapin's analysis of industrial scientists, scientific entrepreneurs, and venture capitalists articulated some of the shifting roles scientists adopted in the late twentieth century and the tensions they faced in an increasingly institutionalized scientific landscape. Throughout it all, Shapin stressed—contrary to the widespread celebration of science as impersonal and the reported demise of the subject—the extraordinary "significance of the personal."[12]

My book has contributed to this discussion about the personal dimensions of science by advancing a rhetorical perspective on the character of scientists and those whose lives are affected by science. My analysis of Datagate has demonstrated how the contests that crop up during controversies that blend technical and public concerns can project, contest, and modify assessments of both the character of science and the character of particular scientists. The emergent rhetorically constituted characters provide proxies for assessing the credibility of expert knowledge. To make this case, I developed a theoretical framework grounded in rhetorical studies with insights from literary theory, science studies, and sociology in order to demonstrate how aspects of character associated with three interwoven but conceptually discrete terms—ethos, persona, and voice—collectively shaped the outcomes, understandings, and preferred policy solutions of the controversy and contributed to the diminishment and eventual restoration of trust. Here, collective assumptions about the normative behavior of scientists (the scientific ethos) prompted recognizable characterizations of individual types of scientists (scientific personae), which, when inflected by an individual scientist's voice, influenced the dynamics, sense-making processes, and policy responses to the controversy.

To scholars of rhetoric and communication studies in particular, this study has demonstrated that the interrelations between the complex and multifaceted characterological concepts of ethos, persona, and voice expose the difficulties of projecting selves through language.[13] The common conflation of ethos, persona, and voice in rhetorical scholarship flattens the horizon of character analysis, discouraging consideration of the multiplicity of characters at the heart of each case. By differentiating between these concepts, we arrive at a fuller appreciation for the link between individuals and communities, between a historical person and their myriad representations in discursive practices, and we can therefore better chart the processes through which character contests animate controversies at the intersection of public, private, and technical life. To date, most examinations of ethos and persona in the rhetoric of science, and many in rhetoric more broadly, have assumed the presence of a single monolithic persona or ethos rather than exploring the interaction of multiple representations of identity.[14] Moreover, these studies have tended to focus on the scientist-rhetor's projection of self rather than to consider the collective, ensemble-like process of character contestation. Countering this tendency, my book has advanced an innovative theoretical perspective on the complexity of character constitution, which has methodological implications for future studies. Here, character can transcend its narrow association with ethos to become a set of multifaceted composites bound up in history, context, and power relations, which tie together elements of ethos, persona, and voice.

To rhetoricians of science, science studies scholars, and stakeholders of science and medicine, this book has offered a contoured map of a credibility contest in a science-related controversy in which competing scientific personae, each embedded in its own narrative universe, vied for dominance in professional, political, and public spheres. The winner of the contest, the persona that resonated most widely, could more strongly influence the controversy's outcomes, ranging from assignments of guilt and ascriptions of morality to policy changes, than those narratives and personae that were less compelling or less penetrating through the spheres. This book has thus laid a path for linking policy outcomes to the process of characterization. It also offered a baseline set of characters that can emerge during science-based controversy for comparison across other cases, each of which will likely exhibit its own characteristics and unique history.

Looking back on the fraying trust and the yawning gap between scientists, politicians, and citizens that we witnessed during Datagate, we can inquire about the implications of this study for understanding the relationship between rhetoric, science, and publics. Addressing this question, this book concludes by attempting to mold some of the lessons of this controversy into a foundation for future inquiry about the thorny interrelationships between trust and truth, character and knowledge, and science and its stake-holders. I begin by discussing the implications of rhetorically constituted characters for knowledge, identity, and action during science-based controversy. I then offer a modest and preliminary proposal for a recharacterization of the available roles of members of scientific and lay publics. Such a proposal is not a panacea for all of the dilemmas that plague contemporary scientific research integrity, however. Rather, I hope to offer a persuasive case that science and its stakeholders require more engagement, not less; that they require a reinvigorated set of relations geared toward greater involvement and dialogue. While trust, transparency, and public participation have become mantralike in science studies, my book asks us to interrogate how our rhetorical practices foster or inhibit public participation in science.

RHETORIC, TRUST, CHARACTER: IMPLICATIONS FOR IDENTITY, KNOWLEDGE, AND ACTION

Although a large and obvious part of the story of Datagate concerned gender, power, and the rights of medical say-so, to argue that the controversy can be reduced to paternalistic physicians, arrogant administrators, sensationalist media, and women forced (yet again) to submit to medical authority is far too facile. My analysis has instead uncovered the complex, multilayered representations of character that can influence science-based controversy. As Datagate's stakeholders wrangled over issues of trust, truth, and ownership of scientific knowledge, they redrew the boundaries of the controversy, and in the process they projected, fortified, and re-created visions of selves and others. Amid Datagate's multiple, contradictory, and fragmented personae, glimpses of the (often contested) values underwriting science shine forth. This observation explains why Roger Poisson's defense of his misdeeds, resoundingly dismissed by the scientific community, could register with some members of broader publics. His claim that he acted to give women the best possible medical care resonated because a number among us want to believe in a heroic doctor who would put patients before bureaucratic mandates. Yet this observation also helps to explain why Poisson could be so easily excised from the church of science. He aired medical science's warts and wrinkles; he flaunted the rules—even if those rules were themselves crystallizing during the time he altered the facts. That his persona of beneficent healer was so muted by a dominant picture of him as a career-minded researcher-turned-fraud helps to explain his fall from grace and sheds insight into why policy solutions that addressed his concerns were not forthcoming. In short, it was more expedient to excise Poisson as supreme violator of the norms of science than to scrutinize the underlying assumptions of the system. Attacking Poisson's character, and then turning to Fisher's management of Poisson, thus left the broader, much thornier issues of clinical trial structure, participation rules, and access to experimental therapies—the very issues that Poisson flouted—largely unchallenged.

When we track the interrelated and overlapping personae of Roger Poisson and Bernard Fisher and evaluate their capacity to engender trust and persuade others of their credibility, we realize the complexity of the challenges they faced. Poisson's implicit argument that he attempted to alleviate the tension he felt as a healer and researcher by bending trial rules produced disastrous result. The personae of beneficent healer and career-minded researcher-turned-fraud clarified the role tension at the heart of his misdeeds. By contrast to Poisson's dichotomous framing, Fisher struggled to overcome multiple and contradictory representations of his character. The persona of scientific revolutionary confirmed Fisher's iconic status and reinforced the myth of the lone genius. It presented a man who alienated the surgical orthodoxy by questioning their cherished Halstedian principles. The persona of reluctant apologist, however, reinforced the separation between scientists, politicians, and publics and exposed the chasm between the norms of scientific reasoning and those of public sphere deliberation. Here, the public sphere expectation, problematically cultivated by politicians with axes to grind, that Fisher should show profound contrition is cited as the reason for his downfall. In this account Fisher's failure to apologize for his actions confirmed perceptions of his arrogance and defied the expectations of his congressional examiners. Finally, in the interaction between the personae of the beleaguered bureaucrat and that of scientific revolutionary, we see fissures in the revolutionary persona, for the bureaucrat exposes the unforgiving administrative side of science, regulated and managed to the hilt. Far from being a genius who boldly charts new paths, the scientist in charge of a clinical trial in this view becomes a glorified paper pusher. The irony, however, is that given the importance of trust and transparency in an era of bureaucratized science, paper pushing provides a necessary rhetorical trace that can be used to marshal evidence of accountability.

This analysis further exposed both the benefits and the limitations of the knowledge consumer persona, which positioned stakeholders outside of the process of scientific production. In this model, stakeholders relied on scientists to tell them the results of clinical research. And though this normative vision is an ethically desirable requirement for science, more robust participation of affected stakeholders would further alleviate a sense of distance and paternalism. Knowledge partners who sit at the table of science can assist with all aspects of research design and implementation, offering their firsthand expert view of what types of treatment regimens are desirable and possible. This sentiment resonates with Craig Waddell's argument that "the public" must be prepared to participate constructively in the scientific and technological controversies that are becoming increasingly crucial to our nation and our world."[15]

We thus discover that characterization in science-based controversy has implications for identity construction, the acceptance of knowledge claims, and for policy outcomes and action. The characterizations to emerge during Datagate—and I suspect other science-based controversies like it—are first and foremost contested constructions of identity. They enfold particular understandings of the (sometimes overlapping) roles of scientist, physician, citizen, patient, social movement, and advocate—and the relationships that can and do exist between them. As philosopher Lauren Marino has asserted, "When we speak we are not only creating new truth relative to the language games we employ, but we create ourselves"—and in the process frame others.[16] Seen in this light, personae do more than bolster or impair knowledge claims. They also expose underlying assumptions about how identities are understood—or misunderstood—in public life. In implicating identities, the personae of science-based controversy reveal the underlying communal ethos of biomedical science. Although they do not neatly reflect the nuances of individual scientific life, such personae do capture the broad thrust of archetypes drawn from the well of collective impression. By tapping in to deeply ingrained, often tacit social understandings, they organize social experience into recurrent, recognizable patterns. In this way, personae mark the boundaries between good science and bad science, trustworthy science and tainted science, a benevolent doctor and a selfish one, a concerned breast cancer advocate and a frightened patient. Ethicist Sydney Halpern has observed that "members of social groups often find it difficult to put words to their informal customs and norms."[17] Against a set of tacit norms and customs, one of the benefits of analysis of the characterizations that populate particular science-based controversies is that it can help scientists and citizens track the underlying values of science by showing us how scientists are to be—and not to be—as they generate knowledge. Because they represent symbolic condensations of the key communal concerns of an epoch, the personae that emerge during science-based controversy can reveal normative assumptions about science and its relationships to and broader antimonies with publics and stakeholders. Each of my case studies has demonstrated how character contests provided occasions for affirming or challenging aspects of scientific practice, and for accepting or rejecting scientific claims about breast cancer treatment.

In the case of knowledge claims, my analysis has revealed how perceptions of character can transform knowledge—not merely by calling it into question because of the perceived character flaws of those who produce it, but also by disrupting, challenging, or fostering trust in the truth claims of scientists and citizens, hence relegating technical reasoning to the standards of public judgment. This study has demonstrated that the personae of science-based controversy, the rhetorically produced character representations of key players, are therefore imbricated with scientific truth. In moments when shattered trust undermined the foundation of faith in truth claims, stakeholders invoked appeals to character as a means of asserting or resisting the fact of lumpectomy's efficacy for early-stage cancers. Using the meter of public trust as a guide, the integrity of the lumpectomy finding was in question because Poisson altered data and Fisher kept news of Poisson's misdeeds in-house. But using technical standards as a guide—following Fisher's claim that even without Poisson's data the findings in support of lumpectomy held—Fisher's scientific character becomes a possible ground for preserving truth and restoring integrity. In other words, when scientific truth enters public life, technical reasoning can recede against audience assessments of credibility, supporting Aristotle's claim that character carries the day, even in the context of science.[18]

My analysis further confirms as untenable the notion that science alone can settle disputes and suggest policy and action. As the struggle to determine the integrity of NSABP studies during Datagate indicates, when diverse publics and stakeholders participate in science-based controversy, the validity of the facts of science themselves are exposed to contestation. In fact, as science policy scholar Daniel Sarewitz noted, "The organization of science—its methodological and disciplinary diversity; the multiple institutional settings in which it is conducted—make it a remarkably potent catalyst for political dispute."[19] Datagate offers a prime example of this phenomenon, underscoring the relevance of trust and credibility, elements that can be transformed by assessments of the character of scientists and other players in the scientific process. Datagate further exposes the perils of assuming that science knows best, of deciding that problems with data are best handled by scientists alone. However, it also reveals the dangers of democratizing knowledge claims, for the Gordian knot at the center of this controversy was that Poisson's actions, defiant and misguided though they were, did not alter the outcomes of NSABP research. In Datagate we therefore witnessed a clash between the norms of technical reasoning, which deemed that Poisson's falsifications were troubling but did not undermine the original study, and the norms of public sphere reasoning, which deemed that Poisson's falsifications cast doubt on the entire federal research enterprise. One way to bridge this chasm is to reconfigure the roles of the scientist and the citizen to cultivate increased scientific engagement with public values and to promote better scientific understanding in public spheres, a task to which I turn in the next section of this chapter.

Finally, in the case of policy and action, because they are embedded in distinct narrative universes, which open or forestall consideration of broader issues of science in public life, personae imply the rightness or wrongness of particular actions and can therefore limit agency and direct attention to particular facets of scientific life and thereby to particular policy solutions. When the character contests swirling around certain players coalesce into a dominant narrative—say, that Poisson's actions were inexcusable—they can foreclose consideration of the underlying assumptions of the system. When, for example, Poisson's actions were widely condemned and dismissed without reflection, the issues concerning the procedures for eligibility requirements and access to experimental treatments were largely ignored. Moreover, when the norms of research advocates coincided with those of knowledge consumers and the Dark Knight of science, then truth-telling was confirmed as a requirement of science. By contrast, if characterization positions players in ways that explicitly call into question underlying norms, then change that addresses those system problems is more likely. Thus, identifying dominant personae helps us to understand why particular policy outcomes focusing on detecting and punishing individual transgressors resulted from Datagate while those that pushed more meaningful stakeholder involvement did not.

(RE)FIGURING NEW CHARACTERS FOR SCIENTIFIC LIFE

As we have seen, characterizations reflect cultural values and implicit norms about science and shape assessments regarding the status of knowledge claims. However, unmasking the assumptions of these roles reveals how participants may unwittingly script themselves as outsiders to the scientific process rather than as able partners. This observation is not intended to criticize those parties who find themselves wronged by or excluded from research processes. Rather, it is meant to prompt a process of reimagining what these roles can be and to craft them in ways that can intervene meaningfully in jurisdictional and procedural debates over science. As Charles

Alan Taylor has observed, "The cultural configuration that privileges science over and against politics (and other cultural discourses) is fundamentally discursive. To suggest that any hierarchical configuration of practices is a rhetorical construction entails as well that it is subject to alternative construction—a task to which rhetorical critics should set themselves."[20]

Recognizing the chasm between scientists and their stakeholders and publics, philosophers of science, science studies scholars, and practitioners have advanced models of citizen participation in science. Many of these posit some permutation of a politically engaged scientist and a scientifically engaged citizen.[21] While the categories of scientist and citizen are not mutually exclusive, they nevertheless index an ethic of mutual engagement. The scientist-citizen/citizen-scientist and the knowledge partner therefore represent but several figures that can disrupt the cold war separation between science and its stakeholders. This first figure represents the politically engaged scientist who refuses to be seduced by the insular model of science. Instead, the scientist-citizen would actively solicit stakeholder input, approaching his or her task with a mind for public values. This persona would thus directly challenge the perceived disinterestedness of science in that the ends of science would be up for reconsideration.

The figure of the citizen engaged with science acknowledges the crucial link between science and society and the gap between expert and lay knowledge.[22] By answering the call for greater "public engagement" with science and technology, patient advocates, citizen members of science advisory boards, and citizen scientists who assist with knowledge production increasingly represent this figure. Prompting consideration of how to involve broader citizen input into science, James Wilsdon and his colleagues have asked, "How do we reach a situation where scientific 'excellence' is automatically taken to include reflection and wider engagement on social and ethical dimensions?"[23] As this question implies, one way of transcending the separation of science and its stakeholders is to push for models of democratic scientific governance that some academics, activists, and policymakers have called "public engagement" with science. Historically, such engagement has taken many forms, including consensus conferences, European-style science shops, and public sessions designed to allow public inputs into science policy.[24] Wilsdon and his coauthors advocate a model of "upstream engagement" that invites consideration of the broader "public values" underlying science. The concept of "public value" that Wilsdon and his colleagues present derives from a robust conception of scientific governance that prompts questions about the overall benefits of scientific practices, priorities, and procedures to human life and well-being—namely, the sociopolitical ends of science rather than merely the technical details. Considering the "public value" of science thus requires participation and representation of members of various publics in scientific research design, implementation, and planning. As Wilsdon and his colleagues explain,

> Public value also clarifies and deepens the rationale for "upstream" public engagement. Viewed through a public value lens, engagement might no longer be seen as a "brake on progress," but instead as a way of maintaining and renewing the social contract that supports science. Upstream engagement enables society to discuss and clarify the public value of science. It encourages dialogue between scientists and the public to move beyond competing propositions, to a richer discussion of visions and ends. And it reminds scientists of the contribution that public *values* can make to the setting of research priorities and trajectories.[25]

The types of reconfigured relationships between science, its stakeholders, and publics implied by this model have the potential for promoting democratic engagement with matters of science, medicine, and technology by allowing members of various publics to deliberate with scientists and policymakers on matters of mutual interest and by providing mechanisms for ventilating ideas. Such engagement can allow both public *participation* and *representation* in the processes affecting science. It may entail performing engagement with science via collective action and multiple, overlapping identities. When Fran Visco testified before Dingell's Congress that inclusion of patient advocates on NSABP advisory boards might have alerted scientists to public perceptions concerning tainted NSABP data, she reflected the desirability of this sort of partnership and the goals of collective action. Such a reconfiguration of roles can begin to create spaces for a more integrated view of engagement with science. Although many breast cancer advocates have already been serving in this capacity, active involvement in all aspects of research design has yet to reach its full potential. Indeed, in the years since Datagate splashed across the headlines, patient advocacy groups have become even more organized in their efforts to participate in the scientific practices that invariably affect their lives. At the same time, breast cancer has become increasingly more mainstream and commercialized. This tendency has transformed breast cancer politics into spectacles of consumption that do raise money and awareness at the same time they keep most women at the fringes of participation in knowledge production, and they discourage further reflection about the broader systemic issues related to cancer and research about cancer. For example, in their study of patients participating in research decisions in the Netherlands between 2000 and 2003, J. Francisca Caron-Flinterman and her coauthors found that biomedical decision making remains "mainly the territory of experts," suggesting that more work remains to incorporate citizen participation in all aspects of biomedical research.[26]

To be sure, characterization, although a promising beginning, cannot alone bridge the rift between science and stakeholders in contemporary life. Systemic measures designed to foster trust and mutual engagement must continue to be put in place and evaluated for their efficacy. These would require greater transparency in decision making and in enhanced communication of study results and potential problems to affected stakeholders. Nonetheless, this book has demonstrated that trust in an individual scientist entails a wider trust in the ability of scientific institutions to detect inauthenticity, sloppiness, error, and fabrication. This process also requires trust in institutions to promote dialogue about norms and their violations but must transcend the mechanics of mere public relations, entailing redesigning research to more heavily involve public inputs into the planning process. In that sense, the scientist as citizen would work in tandem with the face of the citizen engaged with scientific research.

Regardless of the possibilities and liabilities entailed in such roles, future research should interrogate the implications of the figures of the engaged scientist and the citizen engaged with science. On what conceptions of science and of publics do they rest? Do they engender meaningful participation, or do they merely pay lip service to public values and citizen participation? How can meaningful mutual engagement of scientists and citizens be fostered, critiqued, and revised? What are the barriers to mutual engagement? And how can scholars of rhetoric, science studies, and health communication best contribute to answering these questions?

The trends we saw influencing scientists in Datagate—geographical dispersion, bureaucratization, residual models of insularity—challenge the capacity for building the trust relations necessary for knowledge claims to have legitimacy even as they provide new possibilities for science. In addition to the separation between science and citizens, several other complicating factors jeopardize the delicate web of openness and trust that ideally informs scientific practice and that makes public investment in science possible—notably, privatization, profit, conflicts of interest, and lack of access.[27] Peter Sztompa maintains that "the functional imperative for trust may be even more pressing today than it was in earlier periods in the history of science." The reasons for this, he explains, stem from "the global, supranational scope of science; the transdisciplinary character of much research; the dense networks of cooperation and communication among scholars distant in space and otherwise unfamiliar to each other; the unleashed potential for either malicious uses or inadvertent side-effects of science, resulting in grave risks for masses of people; and finally the huge public funds committed to science."[28] As science continues to become more market-driven, bureaucratized, and dispersed, citizens and scientists alike need to find ways of forging arrangements that can overcome these barriers and further foster trust and transparency.

Rhetorician John Lyne has explained that "the various research specialties of the modern day 'knowledge industry' tend to shield themselves from public judgment by their self-isolating vocabularies and by the territorial claims of expertise."[29] "If rhetoricians can begin to get a sense of the rhetorical practices of these specialties," he argued, "it might be possible to make the discourses of academic knowledge better mesh with the discourses of public life."[30] Datagate's chasm between the insular model of science represented by NSABP's initial response to the controversy, combined with citizens' quests for information and involvement, confirms the need for a productive space wherein citizens and scientists can come together to know together, to reason together, and to influence one another's perceptions of epistemic and ethical claims.[31] When viewed through this lens, it is not hard to suggest that perhaps part of the conflict at the heart of Datagate stemmed from a collective failure of imagination, a failure to regard all stakeholders as worthy participants in an ongoing negotiation of the roles each plays in relation to the other.

Datagate demonstrated how the beneficiaries of science, who sometimes clamor for participation but who frequently find themselves engrossed in busy and richly textured lives, become isolated from the production of science and from its public dissemination, deliberation, and discussion. Herein lies a problem, for science's myriad accomplishments rest on its credibility; they rely on the trust of strangers at once both technologically disconnected from, but entirely crucial for, their health and well-being. When considered together, my three case studies of characterization during Datagate—Poisson, Fisher, and advocates and politicians—testify to the struggles of a particular historical moment when several forces converged to transform breast cancer research from the pages of scientific journals into the light of public scrutiny. Despite their particularities, Datagate's debates are deep emblems of a broader set of cultural contests to make science accountable to varied publics. Although overtly about purity, precision, and truth-telling, these debates are vexed by questions concerning who may participate in scientific decision making, what the relationships between science and its stakeholders should be, and the role of science as a public good. Thus, although this book has focused on three case studies of characterization during one breast cancer research controversy, it more broadly has addressed the enmeshments and estrangements of science and everyday life in our present historical moment.

Ultimately, this book has shown how analysis of the rhetorically constituted characters that animate science-based controversy can contribute to an understanding of the dynamics and meanings of such controversies and can yield insights about the place of science in contemporary life. Given the increasing bureaucratization of science, its integration into everyday life and public policy, and its reliance on tax-payer funding on the one hand, and its parallel commercialization, conflicts of interest, and secrecy on the other, talk of trust and character represents only the beginning of a longer but very important conversation. I have intended my analysis as an invitation for those of us who inhabit this twenty-first-century world wherein science interlaces so snugly with everyday life, for those of us who depend on scientists but are never really sure which science, whose science, we can trust. I have meant it as a call for collaboration that represents the opening strains of future dialogue and reflection about how all of us are affected by and can participate in that glorious—and gloriously messy—set of practices we call science.

Appendix
Chronology of the Controversy

Date	Event
Date	*Event*
1958	NSABP founded
1967	Bernard Fisher becomes chair of NSABP; operations move to Pittsburgh
1977	B-06 "lumpectomy" trial begins patient accrual
1980	Saint-Luc Hospital receives clinical trials grant; Roger Poisson named principal investigator
1985	NSABP publishes five-year B-06 results comparing total mastectomy and lumpectomy in breast cancer treatment in *NEJM*
1986	President Ronald Reagan appoints Fisher to National Cancer Advisory Board
1989	NSABP publishes eight-year B-06 results of randomized clinical trial comparing total mastectomy to lumpectomy in *NEJM*
1990	
June	NSABP investigators discover discrepancy reported in date of surgery on operative report of patient at Saint-Luc during a routine audit of data contributed by Dr. Roger Poisson, head of Cancer Research at Saint-Luc; they suggest a more thorough audit

| September | During the audit, the deputy director of NSABP's Biostatistical Center finds several more anomalies and recommends a more extensive second audit |

1991

January	A three-person NSABP team visits Saint-Luc and finds more discrepancies in record keeping
February	The audit team notifies Fisher of Poisson's data falsifications; Poisson is dismissed from his position as principal investigator at Saint-Luc; Fisher and NSABP notify FDA, NCI, and OSI of Poisson's discrepancies; Poisson admits to falsifying data in a faxed letter to Fisher
March	OSI's Division of Research Integrity decides to conduct a formal investigation since misconduct has already occurred

1992

January	NCI funding of Saint-Luc expires
March	NSABP assures NCI and ORI (successor organization to OSI) that there are no major changes to the published findings when Dr. Poisson's data is eliminated from analysis; ORI reports there is general agreement on the need for reanalysis regardless
December	ORI finishes investigation determining that Poisson falsified 7 percent of data

1993

January	NCI officials urge NSABP to finish reanalysis of all studies to which Poisson contributed patients as soon as possible; they offer expedited review for publication in *Journal of the National Cancer Institute*
February	ORI releases findings of their investigation to Poisson and NSABP
March	Poisson is debarred from receiving federal grants for eight years
April	ORI's finding that Poisson was guilty of scientific misconduct is published in ORI newsletter; Poisson

resigns from all administrative positions at
Saint-Luc

June   ORI findings in the investigation of Roger Poisson
are published in the *Federal Register*

1994

March   *Chicago Tribune* issues front-page report of Poisson's
falsifications, noting NSABP's failure to publish
reanalysis of the fourteen studies to which Poisson
contributed; NCI discovers data discrepancy
in second Montreal hospital; they request that
Dr. Fisher be replaced at the NSABP; Congressman John Dingell calls hearings on the matter

April   Robert Herberman replaces Fisher at NSABP on
an "interim basis"; Congressman Dingell holds first
hearing of the Subcommittee on Oversight and
Investigations to address NSABP breast cancer
research misconduct

May   *New England Journal of Medicine* editors Marcia
Angell and Jerome Kassirer publish an essay sharply
criticizing Fisher, Poisson, and the NCI

June   NSABP submits draft of reanalysis to NCI; Dingell
holds second hearing

July   Fisher files lawsuit against the University of Pittsburgh and the federal government for violation of
due process

August   NSABP executive board joins Fisher in lawsuit
against Pittsburgh

September   ORI begins investigation of scientific misconduct at
Pittsburgh

October   Norman Wolmark replaces Fisher as chair of
NSABP

1997

February   ORI concludes Fisher and University of Pittsburgh
are not guilty of scientific misconduct

August   Fisher withdraws lawsuit from the university; the
                    university apologizes, and Fisher is awarded $2.75
                    million in settlement from Pittsburgh with several
                    hundred thousand dollars from NCI; Fisher is effec-
                    tively cleared of "all wrongdoing"

Notes

INTRODUCTION

1. John Crewdson, "Fraud in Breast Cancer Study: Doctor Lied on Data for Decade," *Chicago Tribune*, March 13, 1994, A1.

2. A fuller account of Poisson's actions appears in the Office of Research Integrity's full report on Roger Poisson in U S. Department of Health and Human Services, Office of Research Integrity, *Investigation Report: St. Luc Hospital NSABP Project*, 1993; hereafter, HHS, *Investigation Report: St. Luc.* Copy on file with author.

3. The "all hell broke loose" quotation was attributed to then NSABP director Dr. Bernard Fisher in Mackenzie Carpenter and Steve Twedt, "Anatomy of a Scandal: Fisher Describes Ordeal as 'Reign of Terror,'" *Pittsburgh Post-Gazette*, December 27, 1994, A6.

4. The NIH consensus statement appears in National Institutes of Health, "Treatment of Early-Stage Breast Cancer," *NIH Consensus Statement Online* 8, no. 6 (1990): 1–19, http://consensus.nih.gov/1990/1990EarlyStageBreastCancer081html.htm (accessed June 29, 2009).

5. The lumpectomy with radiation finding held for stage I and II breast cancers. Although other clinical trials weighed in to the consensus statement, influential research reports included the following NSABP publications: Bernard Fisher et al., "Five-Year Results of a Randomized Clinical Trial Comparing Total Mastectomy With or Without Radiation in the Treatment of Breast Cancer," *New England Journal of Medicine* (hereafter, *NEJM*) 312, no. 11 (1985): 665–73; and Bernard Fisher et al., "Eight-Year Results of a Randomized Clinical Trial Comparing Total Mastectomy and Lumpectomy With or Without Irradiation in the Treatment of Breast Cancer," *NEJM* 320, no. 13 (1989): 822–28.

6. Harmon Eyre, quoted in Kathy A. Fackelmann, "Breast Cancer Research on Trial," *Science News* 145, no. 18 (1994): 282.

7. See Fisher et al., "Five-Year Results" and "Eight-Year Results."

8. For a description of Fisher's stunning fall from grace, read Carpenter and Twedt's four-part *Pittsburgh Post-Gazette* series "Anatomy of a Scandal," and Lawrence K. Altman, "Fall of a Man Pivotal in Breast Cancer Research," *New York Times,* April 3, 1994, B10, http://www.nytimes.com/1994/04/04/us/fall-of-a-man-pivotal-in-breast-cancer-research.html (accessed September 25, 2009). Fisher's continued struggles to clear his name are outlined in Chris B. Pascal, "Misconduct Annotations," *Science* 274, no. 5290 (1996): 1065–69, while his reputational restoration is chronicled in Leah Kauffman, "Bernard Fisher in Conversation," interview, *Pitt Med* 4, no. 3 (July 2002): 12–15, http://pittmed.health.pitt.edu/JUL_2002/feature_BFisher.pdf (accessed July 1, 2009).

9. Bernard Fisher et al., "Reanalysis and Results after 12 Years of Follow-up in a Randomized Clinical Trial Comparing Total Mastectomy With Lumpectomy With or Without Irradiation in the Treatment of Breast Cancer," *NEJM* 333 (1995): 1456–61; and Anita Srikameswaran, "20-Year Study Shows Lumpectomies Work," *Pittsburgh Post-Gazette,* October 17, 2002, www.post-gazette.com/healthscience/20021017breast1017P2.asp (accessed September 23, 2009).

10. I extracted these figures from HHS, *Investigation Report: St. Luc.*

11. Ibid.

12. Breast cancer survivor and journalist Roberta K. Altman coined the descriptor "NSABP Datagate" in *Waking Up, Fighting Back: The Politics of Breast Cancer* (New York: Little, Brown, 1996), 184. I recognize that the act of naming is political and decided to use the abbreviated form of Altman's moniker, "Datagate," because it does not link the controversy to a specific person, unlike other possible names such as "*L'Affaire Poisson*" or "the Fisher controversy." My use of this label is not intended to imply intentional cover-up. Rather, I believe the problems of Datagate resulted from multiple misunderstandings and different presumptions about the obligations of science.

13. Rayna Rapp, "Accounting for Amniocentesis," in *Knowledge, Power, and Practice: The Anthropology of Health,* ed. S. Lindenbaum and M. Lock (Berkeley: University of California Press, 1993), 63.

14. My use of the term *science-based controversy* throughout the book indexes the mix of public and technical concerns that occurs in this and many other publicly contested cases concerning science. For further work on science-based controversies, see Thomas Brante, "Reasons for Studying Scientific and Scientific-Based Controversies," in *Controversial Science: From Content to Contention,* ed. Thomas Brante, Steve Fuller, and W. Lynch (Albany: SUNY Press), 177–92; Josh Boyd, "Public and Technical Interdependence: Regulatory Controversy, Out-law Discourse, and the Messy Case of Olestra," *Argumentation and Advocacy* 39 (2002): 91–109; and Lisa Keränen, "Mapping Misconduct: Demarcating Legitimate Science from 'Fraud' in the B-06 Lumpectomy Study," *Argumentation and Advocacy* (2005): 94–113.

15. John Hardwig, "The Role of Trust in Knowledge," *Journal of Philosophy* 88 (1991): 702.

16. Walter J. Ong, "Voice as a Summons for Belief," in *The Barbarian Within and Other Fugitive Essays and Studies* (New York: Macmillan, 1962), 91–92.

17. Arnold S. Relman, quoted in the opening epigraph of Carl Djerassi's novel about research misconduct, *Cantor's Dilemma* (New York: Penguin Books, 1989), n.p.

18. See University of Pittsburgh, "Fisher Drops Suit in Exchange for Apology, $2.75 Million; University Administrators Credited with Bringing About Settlement," *University Times* 30, no. 2, September 11, 1997, http://tinyurl.com/p8l3ca (accessed June 30, 2009); and "Public Statement Incidental to Termination of Litigation in RE: Fisher vs. University of Pittsburgh et al.," *University Times* 30, no. 2, September 11, 1997, http://tinyurl.com/lh6upb (accessed June 30, 2009). For Fisher's reply, see University of Pittsburgh, "Bernard Fisher," *University Times* 30, no. 2, September 11, 1997, http://tinyurl.com/pjt6ww (accessed June 30, 2009).

19. Stephen Hilgartner, *Science on Stage: Expert Advice as Public Drama* (Stanford, CA: Stanford University Press, 2000).

20. The canonical essay concerning spheres of argument is G. Thomas Goodnight, "The Personal, Technical, and Public Spheres of Argument: A Speculative Inquiry into the Art of Public Deliberation," *Journal of the American Forensic Association* 18 (1982): 214–27.

21. The scope of rhetoric has been a much-debated topic, particularly during the twentieth century (see, for one example commenting on this topic, Donald C. Bryant, "Rhetoric: Its Functions and Its Scope," *Quarterly Journal of Speech* 39 [1953]: 401–24). While rhetoric's revival in the early decades of the twentieth century often featured political oratory and orators, later years broadened the scope of rhetoric to include any symbol use. By the 1970s, rhetoricians were studying protest rhetoric, film, and even the rhetoric of science. Helpful overviews of the trajectory of rhetorical scholarship can be found in William L. Nothstine, Carole Blair, and Gary A. Copeland, "Invention in Media and Rhetorical Criticism: A General Orientation," in *Critical Questions: Invention, Creativity, and the Criticism of Discourse and Media,* ed. William L. Nothstine, Carole Blair, and Gary A. Copeland (New York: St. Martin's, 1994), 3–14; and William L. Nothstine, Carole Blair, and Gary A. Copeland, "Professionalization and the Eclipse of Critical Invention," in *Critical Questions,* 15–63.

22. A review of various positions on the relationship between rhetoric and scientific truth, including the view that rhetoric is constitutive of scientific facts, appears in Alan G. Gross, *Starring the Text: The Place of Rhetoric in Science Studies* (Carbondale: Southern Illinois University Press, 2006).

23. I am aware of divergent literatures and connotations regarding *stakeholders* and *publics,* but here I use the terms nearly interchangeably to refer to those persons with a vested interest in the outcomes of the issues at hand. Sometimes the term *stakeholders* refers to specific collectivities involved with a particular issue while *publics* connotes those involved in a broader dialogue. Moreover, I want to stress that the terms *scientist* and *citizen* simplify the complex subject positions and relations of each and are not mutually exclusive. Substitute terms like *lay experts* only compli-

cate matters, but I do want to acknowledge the multiplicity and overlapping nature of positions and roles regarding citizens and science.

24. S. Michael Halloran, "The Birth of Molecular Biology: An Essay in the Rhetorical Criticism of Scientific Discourse," in *Landmark Essays on Rhetoric of Science: Case Studies*, Landmark Essays Series, vol. 11., ed. Randy Allen Harris (Mahwah, NJ: Lawrence Erlbaum, 1997), 48.

25. James T. Patterson, *The Dread Disease: Cancer and Modern American Culture* (Cambridge, MA: Harvard University Press, 1987).

26. NSABP, "NSABP Timeline," http://www.nsabp.pitt.edu/NSABP_Timeline .pdf (accessed July 2, 2009). Conflicting dates ranging from 1957 to 1967 for the founding of NSABP and for Fisher's installation of it in Pittsburgh appear in various medical journals and newspaper accounts.

27. NSABP is characterized as "perhaps America's most esteemed breast cancer research group" by Steve Austin and Cathy Hitchcock, *Breast Cancer: What You Should Know (But May Not Be Told) about Prevention, Diagnosis, and Treatment* (Rocklin, CA: Prima, 1994), 40, quoted in George Goldberg, *Enough Already! The Overtreatment of Early Breast Cancer* (Tucson, AZ: Paracelsus Press, 1996), 62.

28. Fisher et al., "Five-Year Results," and "Eight-Year Results."

29. HHS, *Investigation Report: St. Luc*, 3.

30. One NSABP investigator told me under conditions of anonymity that he learned of the problems with NSABP trial data one evening when listening to National Public Radio years after NSABP had discovered them. He described his reaction as "flabbergasted."

31. Poisson's misdeeds are recounted in HHS, *Investigation Report: St. Luc*.

32. NIH, "Treatment of Early-Stage Breast Cancer."

33. HHS, *Investigation Report: St. Luc*.

34. When the controversy began, the Office of Science Integrity (OSI) was charged with overseeing the investigation. In 1993 OSI underwent a structural reorganization that collapsed two offices, the OSI and the Office of Scientific Integrity Review (OSIR), into the Office of Research Integrity (ORI). See HHS, *Investigation Report: St. Luc*.

35. See "Findings of Scientific Misconduct," *Federal Register* 58, no. 117 (1993): 33831.

36. Kathy Sawyer, "Cancer Researcher's Credibility Ailing; Exposure of Surgeon's 13-Year Deception Has Heavy Public Impact," *Washington Post*, April 13, 1994, A1.

37. Carpenter and Twedt, "Scandal: Fisher Describes Ordeal," A1.

38. Pascal, "Misconduct Annotations."

39. These concerns aired in the months prior to the Datagate controversy. See Fran Visco, "Testimony of Fran Visco, President, National Breast Cancer Coalition," U.S. House of Representatives, Subcommittee on Oversight and Investigations of the Committee on Energy and Commerce, *Scientific Misconduct in Breast Cancer*

Research, 103rd Cong., 2nd sess., April 13 and June 15 (Washington, DC: U.S. Government Printing Office, 1994) (hereafter, U.S. House, *Scientific Misconduct*), 18. Full text available at http://www.archive.org/stream/scientificmiscon00unit/ scientificmiscon00unit_djvu.txt (accessed July 1, 2009).

40. Eliot Marshall, "Tamoxifen: Hanging in the Balance," *Science* 264, no. 5165 (1994): 1524.

41. Carpenter and Twedt, "Scandal: Fisher Describes Ordeal," A1.

42. Ibid., A6. Some administrators did in fact know about the problems. ORI sent the University of Pittsburgh's research integrity officers a copy of their final report on the Poisson affair in February 1993, while deans George Bernier and Donald Mattison informed Fisher in May 1993 that an inquiry would be conducted on the matter of his alleged knowing use of falsified data in NSABP publications, according to HHS, *Investigation Report: St. Luc,* 13.

43. Carpenter and Twedt, "Scandal: Fisher Describes Ordeal," A1.

44. Ibid.

45. Ibid.

46. Ibid.

47. Kirsten Boyd Goldberg and Paul Goldberg, eds., "Fisher Unable to Answer Key Questions; Blames NCI at Second Hearing on NSABP," *Cancer Letter* 20, no. 25 (1994): 2.

48. Steve Twedt, "Data Problems Cited at 11 Cancer Centers," *Pittsburgh Post-Gazette,* June 16, 1994, A12.

49. Ibid.

50. Ibid.

51. Goldberg and Goldberg, "Fisher Unable to Answer," 1.

52. Jill Lea Sigal, "Testimony of Jill Sigal, Consultant," U.S. House, *Scientific Misconduct,* 29.

53. Daniel S. Greenberg, "Dingell and the Breast Cancer Trials," *Lancet* 343, no. 8905 (1994): 1089.

54. Sigal testimony, U.S. House, *Scientific Misconduct,* 29.

55. Ibid.

56. "Breast Cancer Study Fraud," *ABC World News Sunday,* transcript #411, March 13, 1994.

57. Harmon Eyre, quoted in Sheryl Stolberg, "Feeling Betrayed by Science; A Scandal over Faked Data in a Breast Cancer Study Has Left Patients Reeling and a Pioneering Doctor in Disgrace," *Los Angeles Times,* April 1, 1994, A22.

58. See Wade Roush, "John Dingell: Dark Knight of Science," *Technology Review* 95 (January 1992): 58; John Dingell, quoted in Bruce Bimber and David H. Guston, "Politics by the Same Means: Government and Science in the United States," in *Handbook of Science and Technology Studies,* ed. Sheila Jasanoff et al. (Thousand Oaks, CA: Sage, 1995), 566.

59. Rick Weiss, "NIH: The Price of Neglect," *Science* 251, no. 4993 (1991):

508–11. The term *big science,* attributed to physicist Alvin Weinberg, refers to the large-scale, multisite, multi-investigator, government-funded research installed in laboratories or universities during and after World War II. See Alvin M. Weinberg, "Impact of Large-Scale Science on the United States," *Science* 134, no. 3473 (1961): 161–64.

60. John Dingell statement, U.S. House, *Scientific Misconduct,* 101.

61. I keep emphasizing "women" because most breast cancer cases strike women. According to the American Cancer Society's Web site (www.cancer.org), approximately two hundred thousand cases of breast cancer are diagnosed in the United States each year. Only 1 percent of these cases involve men. Also, as I shall detail in chapter 4, obviously not all women responded with alarm.

62. HHS, *Investigation Report: St. Luc,* 37.

63. "What Is Truth?" editorial, *Lancet* 343, no. 8911 (1994): 1443.

64. Kirsten Boyd Goldberg and Paul Goldberg, "Second Irregularity in NSABP Data Found; Fisher Takes Leave as Group's Chairman," *Cancer Letter* 20, no. 13 (1994): 3.

65. Christine Gorman, "Breast Cancer: A Diagnosis of Deceit," *Time,* June 24, 2001, 52.

66. Sigal testimony, U.S. House, *Scientific Misconduct,* 29.

67. Benedict Carey, "Criticism of a Gender Theory, and a Scientist under Siege," *New York Times,* August 21, 2007, http://www.nytimes.com/2007/08/21/health/psychology/21gender.html?_r=1&oref=slogin (accessed June 30, 2009); Robert Lee Hotz, "Most Science Studies Appear to Be Tainted by Sloppy Analysis," *Wall Street Journal,* September 14, 2007, B1; and Will Dunham, "Health Researchers Cleared of Vaccine Misconduct," Reuter's News, September 28, 2007, http://www.reuters.com/article/domesticNews/idUSN2845456620070928 (accessed July 2, 2009).

68. Judy Segal and Alan Richardson, "Introduction: Scientific Ethos: Authority, Authorship, and Trust in the Sciences," *Configurations* 11, no. 2 (2003): 139.

69. This book offers a study of character, not of apologetic discourse per se, although the two are closely related and scientists and oversight officials sometimes use the genre in efforts at image restoration. For insight into the robust tradition of research concerning apologiae, see B. L. Ware and Wil A. Linkugel, "They Spoke in Defense of Themselves: On the Generic Criticism of Apologia," *Quarterly Journal of Speech* 59 (1973): 273–83; Halford Ross Ryan, "Kategoria and Apologia: On Their Rhetorical Criticism as a Speech Set," *Quarterly Journal of Speech* 68 (1982): 254–61, and his edited *Oratorical Encounters: Selected Studies and Sources of Twentieth-Century Political Accusations and Apologies* (New York: Greenwood Press, 1988); and Martin Carcasson and James Arnt Aune, "Klansman on the Court: Justice Hugo Black's 1937 Radio Address," *Quarterly Journal of Speech* 89 (2003): 154–70.

70. Yaron Ezrahi, "The Political Resources of American Science," *Science Studies* 1, no. 2 (1971): 117. See also Susan E. Cozzens and Edward J. Woodhouse, "Science, Government, and the Politics of Knowledge," in *Handbook of Science and Technology Studies,* ed. Jasanoff et al.

CHAPTER 1

1. Goldberg and Goldberg, "Second Irregularity," 3. The irregularity, concerning a date on a chart, was found at Montreal's St. Mary's Hospital, which was affiliated with McGill University.

2. Ibid.

3. Ibid.

4. Gordon R. Mitchell, *Strategic Deception: Rhetoric, Science and Politics in Missile Defense Advocacy* (East Lansing: Michigan State University Press, 2000).

5. Richard Rorty, "Science as Solidarity," in *Objectivity, Relativism, and Truth* (New York: Cambridge University Press, 1991), 35.

6. Ibid.

7. Brian Martin, "Strategies for Dissenting Scientists," *Journal of Scientific Exploration* 12, no. 4 (1998): 605–16, http://www.uow.edu.au/arts/sts/bmartin/pubs/98jse.html (accessed July 1, 2009).

8. Daniel Patrick Thurs, *Science Talk: Changing Notions of Science in American Popular Culture* (New Brunswick, NJ: Rutgers University Press, 2007), 111.

9. Steven Shapin, *The Scientific Life: A Moral History of a Late Modern Vocation* (Chicago: University of Chicago Press, 2008), 3.

10. Thomas F. Gieryn, *Cultural Boundaries of Science: Credibility on the Line* (Chicago: University of Chicago Press, 1999), 1.

11. Ibid.

12. My essay "Mapping Misconduct" demonstrates how dominant framings of science-based controversies push particular policy outcomes, which can reconfigure the bounds of legitimate scientific practice. See Keränen, "Mapping Misconduct."

13. Harriet Zuckerman, "Deviant Behavior and Social Control in Science," in *Deviance and Social Change,* ed. E. Sagarin (Beverly Hills, CA: Sage, 1977), 127.

14. David Lindsay Watson, *Scientists Are Human* (London: Watts, 1938).

15. Ibid., 21.

16. Rhetoricians will recognize the Aristotelian flavor of this formulation as seen in *The Rhetoric and the Poetics of Aristotle,* trans. W. R. Roberts and I. Bywater (New York: Modern Library, 1984). For divergent perspectives on ethos, see Charles Chamberlain, "From 'Haunts' to 'Character': The Meaning of Ethos and Its Relation to Ethics," *Helios* 11, no. 2 (1984): 97–108; Helen Constantinides, "The Duality of Scientific Ethos: Deep and Surface Structures," *Quarterly Journal of Speech* 87 (2001): 61–72; Ruth Amossy, "Ethos at the Crossroads of Disciplines: Rhetoric, Pragmatics, Sociology," *Poetics Today* 22 (2001): 1–23; James S. Baumlin and Tita F. Baumlin, eds., *Ethos: New Essays in Rhetorical and Critical Theory* (Dallas: Southern Methodist University Press, 1994); and Michael J. Hyde, "Rhetorically, We Dwell," in *The Ethos of Rhetoric,* ed. Michael J. Hyde (Columbia: University of South Carolina Press, 2004), xiii–xxviii.

17. It is important to acknowledge that earlier rhetorical treatments of science

appear in Kenneth Burke, *Counter-Statement* (Berkeley: University of California Press, 1968); and Richard M. Weaver, *The Ethics of Rhetoric* (1953; Davis, CA: Hermagoras Press, 1985). For an overview of exemplary scholarship in the rhetoric of science, see R. Harris, *Landmark Essays on Rhetoric of Science.* Other notable books that introduce readers to this topic include Charles Bazerman, *Shaping Written Knowledge: The Genre and Activity of the Experimental Article in Science* (Madison: University of Wisconsin Press, 1988); Gross, *Starring the Text;* Leah Ceccarelli, *Shaping Science with Rhetoric: The Cases of Dobzhansky, Schrödinger, and Wilson* (Chicago: University of Chicago Press, 2001); Lawrence J. Prelli, *A Rhetoric of Science: Inventing Scientific Discourse* (Columbia: University of South Carolina Press, 1989); and Herbert W. Simons, ed., *The Rhetorical Turn: Invention and Persuasion in the Conduct of Inquiry* (Chicago: University of Chicago Press, 1990). Judy Z. Segal offers a landmark book on the rhetoric of medicine as a subset of the rhetoric of science in *Health and the Rhetoric of Medicine* (Carbondale: Southern Illinois University Press, 2006).

18. R. Harris, introduction to *Landmark Essays on Rhetoric of Science,* xii.

19. Charles Alan Taylor, *Defining Science: A Rhetoric of Demarcation* (Madison: University of Wisconsin Press, 1996), 15.

20. The view that rhetoric is epistemic—that is, that rhetoric is implicated in knowing—is most cogently expressed in Robert L. Scott, "On Viewing Rhetoric as Epistemic," *Central States Speech Journal* 18 (1967): 9–17. However, the idea is as old as the sophists; Protagoras, for instance, is attributed with the maxim "Man is the measure of all things," which posits a human and rhetorical view of knowledge. Scott's view of rhetoric as epistemic has been debated; c.f., Barry Brummett, "The Reported Demise of Epistemic Rhetoric: A Eulogy for Epistemic Rhetoric," *Quarterly Journal of Speech* 76 (1990): 69–72.

21. For introductions to science studies, see David Hess, *Science Studies: An Advanced Introduction* (New York: NYU Press, 1997); Mario Biagioli, ed. *The Science Studies Reader* (New York: Routledge, 1999); and John Ziman, *An Introduction to Science Studies: The Philosophical and Social Aspects of Science and Technology* (New York: Cambridge University Press, 1984).

22. Taylor, *Defining Science,* 6.

23. Celeste Condit, "Contributions of the Rhetorical Perspective to the Social Placement of Medical Genetics," *Communication Studies* 46 (1995): 119.

24. Scott, "On Viewing Rhetoric," 9. Rhetoricians debate whether science is reducible to rhetoric. I believe that it is not. See Gross, *Starring the Text,* for a review of this debate.

25. Prelli, *Rhetoric of Science,* 14.

26. Nothstine, Blair, and Copeland, "Invention in Media," 3.

27. Richard Harvey Brown, *Toward a Democratic Science: Scientific Narration and Civic Communication* (New Haven, CT: Yale University Press, 1998), 106. Some of the quotations concerning rhetorical constructions of character that appear in this chapter were also used in Lisa Keränen, "Competing Characters in Science-Based

Controversy: A Framework for Analysis," in *Understanding Science: New Agendas in Communication,* ed. LeeAnn Kahlor and Patricia Stout (New York: Routledge, 2010): 133–60.

28. Shapin, *Scientific Life,* 311.

29. James S. Ettema and Theodore L. Glasser, "Narrative Form and Moral Force: The Realization of Innocence and Guilt through Investigative Journalism," *Journal of Communication* 38, no. 2 (1988): 8–26; reprinted in *Methods of Rhetorical Criticism: A Twentieth-Century Perspective,* 3rd ed., ed. Bernard L. Brock, Robert L. Scott, and James W. Chesebro (Detroit: Wayne State University Press, 1989), 256.

30. Ibid., 257.

31. Hayden White, quoted in ibid., 258.

32. Marshall W. Alcorn Jr., "Self-Structure as a Rhetorical Device: Modern Ethos and the Divisiveness of the Self," in *Ethos: New Essays in Rhetorical and Critical Theory,* ed. J. S. Baumlin and T. F. Baumlin (Dallas: Southern Methodist University Press, 1994), 3, emphasis in original. Roger Cherry offers two thought-provoking essays concerning the relationship between ethos and persona: "Ethos Versus Persona," *Written Communication* 5 (1988): 251–76; and "Ethos Versus Persona: Self-Representation in Written Discourse," *Written Communication* 15 (1998): 384–410.

33. Aristotle defines the artistic proofs in 1355b-1356a of *Rhetoric.* This particular quotation, however, comes from 1366a, when Aristotle discusses praise and blame.

34. Nan Johnson, "Ethos," in *Encyclopedia of Rhetoric and Composition: Communication from Ancient Times to the Information Age,* ed. Theresa Enos (New York: Garland, 1996), 243.

35. Carolyn R. Miller and S. Michael Halloran, "Reading Darwin, Reading Nature; or, On the Ethos of Historical Science," in *Understanding Scientific Prose,* ed. Jack Selzer (Madison: University of Wisconsin Press, 1993), 121.

36. Aristotle, *Rhetoric;* S. Michael Halloran, "Aristotle's Concept of Ethos; or If Not His, Somebody Else's," *Rhetoric Review* 1, no. 1 (1982): 60.

37. Aristotle, *Rhetoric,* 1356a.

38. Ibid.

39. N. Johnson, "Ethos," 243.

40. Aristotle, *Rhetoric,* 1355b. Also, a speaker whose speech demonstrates the three qualities of ethos that Aristotle enumerates, *phronesis, arête,* and *eunoia*—good sense, good moral character, and goodwill—is persuasive to auditors, for these are the three things people trust besides logical demonstration. See *Rhetoric,* 1378a. See also Eugene Garver, *Aristotle's Rhetoric: An Art of Character* (Chicago: University of Chicago Press, 1994).

41. Isocrates stressed the importance of character development outside of the speaking situation. He wrote: "The man who wishes to persuade people will not be negligent as to the matter of character [ethos]; no, on the contrary, he will apply himself above all to establish a most honorable name among his fellow-citizens;

for who does not know that words carry greater conviction when spoken by men of good repute than when spoken by men who live under a cloud, and that the argument which is made by a man's life is more weight than that which is furnished by words?" In *Antidosis*, trans. George Norlin (Cambridge, MA: Harvard University Press, 1982), 278.

42. Hyde, *Ethos of Rhetoric,* xxiv.

43. Chamberlain, "From 'Haunts' to 'Character,'" 97.

44. Ibid., 97.

45. Ibid., 101.

46. Ibid., 102.

47. Robert K. Merton, "The Normative Structure of Science," in *The Sociology of Science: Theoretical and Empirical Investigations,* ed. Norman K. Storer (Chicago: University of Chicago Press, 1973), 268–69.

48. Merton's thoughts on the ethos of science originally appeared in "A Note on Science and Democracy," *Journal of Legal and Political Sociology* 1 (1942): 115–26. Most readers first encounter the reprint of this essay, titled, "The Normative Structure of Science," in Storer's edited *Sociology of Science,* 254–66. Stephen Turner offers an excellent review of the international scientific and political climate in which Merton produced his ideas in "Merton's Norms in Political and Intellectual Context," *Journal of Classical Sociology* 7 (2007): 161–78. Turner's essay is but one of a series of articles on Merton's norms that appear in the volume.

49. See Ziman, *Introduction to Science Studies.*

50. Sheila Jasanoff, "Contested Boundaries in Policy-Relevant Science," *Social Studies of Science* 17 (1987): 196.

51. Robert Alan Brookey, "Persona," in *Encyclopedia of Rhetoric,* ed. Thomas O. Sloane (New York: Oxford University Press, 2001), 569.

52. Ibid. A number of rhetorical scholars have transcended the literary use of the term *persona* to designate, not a rhetor, but an audience constructed by a text, thus proffering a creative and generative but nonetheless distinct turn away from earlier uses of the term. Examples of this tendency include Edwin Black's second persona as the audience constructed by a text, Philip Wander's third persona as the audience neglected by a text, and Chuck Morris's fourth persona as the audience silenced by the text. By contrast, Paul Campbell's pioneering but somewhat neglected 1975 *Quarterly Journal of Speech* article, "The *Personae* of Scientific Discourse," maintains that scientific discourse has a distinct persona. However, Campbell's use of the term *persona* does not provide space for consideration of how particular scientists can both adhere to a scientific ethos at the same time that they forge distinct personae as scientists. Although these treatments of personae are analytically heuristic, they diverge from the sense of persona I want to rehabilitate, which conceives persona as a recurrent role emergent from cultural stereotypes, a sort of stock public image that is widely recognizable, that audiences use in assessing the ethos of individual players in controversy, and that derives from a more collective sense of ethos as communal

dwelling place. See Edwin Black, "The Second *Persona*," *Quarterly Journal of Speech* 56 (1970): 109; Philip Wander, "The Third Persona: An Ideological Turn in Rhetorical Criticism," *Central States Speech Journal* 35 (1984): 197–216; and Charles E. Morris III, "Pink Herring and the Fourth Persona: J. Edgar Hoover's Sex Crime Panic," in *Readings in Rhetorical Criticism*, 3rd ed., ed. Carl Burgchardt (State College, PA: Strata, 2005), 664–82.

53. Jim W. Corder, "Hunting for *Ethos* Where They Say It Can't Be Found," *Rhetoric Review* 7 (1989): 312.

54. Marcel Mauss speculated that the term may actually have Etruscan origins (*porsenna*) in *Une Catégorie de L'espirit Humain: La Notion de Personne, celle de "Moi"* [A Category of the Human Mind: The Notion of the Person, the Notion of the "Self"] (1939; London: Huxley, 1979).

55. R. C. Elliott, *The Literary Persona* (Chicago: University of Chicago Press, 1982), 21.

56. Mauss, *Catégorie de L'espirit Humain*, 78.

57. W. Martin Bloomer, "Schooling in Persona: Imagination and Subordination in Roman Education," *Classical Antiquity* 16 (1997): 57–78.

58. Ibid., 59.

59. Mauss's *Catégorie de L'esprit Humain* illuminates the cultural role of personae by tracing the shift from *personnage*, or role, in Greek, Roman, Indian, and indigenous cultures to the emergence of self, "*moi*," in the eighteenth century in European Christian cultures.

60. Walker Gibson, quoted in Paul Newell Campbell, "The Personae of Scientific Discourse," *Quarterly Journal of Speech* 61 (1975): 394, emphasis added to Gibson's words by Campbell. Gibson's work is *Persona: A Style Study for Readers and Writers*. New York: Random House, 1969.

61. B. L. Ware and Wil A. Linkugel, "The Rhetorical Persona: Marcus Garvey as Black Moses," *Communication Monographs* 49 (1982): 51.

62. John Lyne and Henry F. Howe, "'Punctuated Equilibrium': Rhetorical Dynamics of a Scientific Controversy," *Quarterly Journal of Speech* 72 (1986): 143. Judy Segal and Alan Richardson identify the dense mix of relationships involved in personae. These include "the relation of the character of science to the character of those who perform it, the means by which the character of science is represented in the *personae* of individual speaker-scientists, and the ways in which the community of scientists is linked to the larger society by virtue of shared values instantiated in the character of science." All of these are implicated in the co-construction of characters in science-based controversy. See Segal and Richardson, "Introduction: Scientific Ethos," 137.

63. Francesca Bordogna, "Scientific Personae in American Psychology: Three Case Studies," *Studies in the History and Philosophy of Biology and the Biomedical Sciences* 36 (2005): 96.

64. Jacob Bronowski is the author of the 1965 treatise *Science and Human Values*.

Theodore Roszak is the author of *The Making of Counter Culture* (1969), which includes an attack on the "deep personality structure of the ideal scientist" as cited in P. Campbell, "Personae of Scientific Discourse," 397.

65. Richard M. Weaver discusses the inherently positive meanings a culture associates with god-terms in his *Ethics of Rhetoric;* Kenneth Burke does the same in *The Rhetoric of Religion: Studies in Logology* (Berkeley: University of California Press, 1961) and *Language as Symbolic Action* (Berkeley: University of California Press, 1968). For instance, in Western culture, *freedom* and *democracy* are god-terms.

66. Ware and Linkugel, "Rhetorical Persona," 50.

67. Ong, "Voice as a Summons," 54.

68. Kenneth Zagacki and William Keith, "Rhetoric, *Topoi,* and Scientific Revolutions," *Philosophy and Rhetoric* 25 (1992): 59–78. Lyne and Howe discuss persona in "Punctuated Equilibria," and of course, Campbell considers it extensively in "Personae of Scientific Discourse."

69. Peter Elbow, "Introduction: About Voice and Writing," in *Landmark Essays on Voice and Writing,* ed. Peter Elbow (Mahwah, NJ: Hermagoras Press, 1994), xx. In "'Voice' and 'Voicelessness' in Rhetorical Studies," Eric King Watts similarly reviewed the conflicting senses of voice that located it either in a speaker or in his or her larger community. He explained, "As it stands now, 'voice' is an ambiguous and redundant concept. It is another term for the 'speaking' subject. It represents the vocabulary of an interpretive community. It is a synonym of style. It is a catchall term that means too many things." *Quarterly Journal of Speech* 87 (2001): 185. Watts also noted more than one hundred essays concerning voice in the rhetorical corpus that exhibited these varied senses.

70. Watts, "'Voice' and 'Voicelessness.'"

71. Elbow, "About Voice and Writing," xxi.

72. Ibid., xxviii–xxxix.

73. Ibid., xxxix.

74. Rhetorician Tom Lessl argues that scientists speak with a priestly voice, "on behalf of an elite subgroup of society (in the case of science a cognitive subculture)," which "bears the responsibility for making its esoteric concepts meaningful without overreaching the linguistic limits of an initiate audience." "The Priestly Voice," *Quarterly Journal of Speech* 75 (1989): 185.

75. Amossy, "Ethos at the Crossroads," 2.

76. Pierre Bourdieu, *Language and Symbolic Power,* trans. G. Raymondson and M. Adamson (Cambridge, UK: Polity Press, 1991), 109.

77. Ibid.

78. In contemporary rhetorical theory (as opposed to cultural or social theory), the pragmatic, instrumentalist, or Aristotelian sense of ethos seems to have prevailed over Platonic or poststructural ones with a few notable (and in the years since I started writing this book, increasingly prominent) exceptions. See, for example, Christian Lundberg and Joshua Gunn, "'Ouija Board, Are There Any Communications?' Agency, Ontotheology, and the Death of the Humanist Subject; or, Con-

tinuing the ARS Conversation," *Rhetoric Society Quarterly* 35 (2005): 83–105, for a critique of the humanist conception of agency, and Weaver, *Ethics of Rhetoric,* for a Platonic vision. Many rhetoric of science scholars either explicitly or implicitly adopt an Aristotelian conception of ethos as the character of the speaker that is linguistically forged through the rhetor's inventional choices. Mark Runquist's analysis of ethos in the writings of American geologists, for example, treats ethos as "the representation of the author in the text and the appeals he/she makes that show the work represents *good* science." See Mark Runquist, "The Rhetoric of Geology: Ethos in the Writing of North American Geologists, 1823–1988," *Journal of Technical Writing and Communication* 22, no. 4 (1992): 388. Lawrence Prelli's conception of scientific ethos similarly concerns "how an audience perceives the professional character of a scientific rhetor or a group of rhetors" and appears in *Rhetoric of Science,* 105. More recently, Helen Constantinides seeks to expand the Aristotelian notion of ethos, noting that "inasmuch as Aristotle's more explicit definitions of *ethos* are found inadequate, *ethos* in the scientific forum is reduced to a vague sense of credibility." See Constantinides, "Duality of Scientific Ethos," 61. Constantinides attempts to refine the Aristotelian sense of ethos by augmenting it with Noam Chomsky's theory of deep and surface structure. Thus, she argues for a dual sense of ethos residing in both the surface structure of style and the deep structure of argument. There are several problems with the apparent flattening of the term ethos that Constantinides identifies. First, audiences seldom share uniform assessments of a speaker's ethos. Second, this perspective underemphasizes how the constructedness of a self through language and its embeddedness in a communal dwelling place results from a linguistic process involving multiple rhetors engaged in a character contest. For another study of ethos in science, see Carolyn R. Miller, "Technology as a Form of Consciousness: A Study of Contemporary Ethos," *Central States Speech Journal* 29 (1978): 228–36.

79. Ware and Linkugel, "Rhetorical Persona," 50.

80. Although there are undoubtedly different personae in specific scientific specialties, because participants in Datagate collapsed them all under the label of "scientists," I follow their cue.

81. Vannevar Bush, *Science—The Endless Frontier: A Report to the President* (Washington, DC: U.S. Government Printing Office, 1945), 19.

82. Marcel C. LaFollette, "The Pathology of Research Fraud: The History and Politics of the U.S. Experience," *Journal of Internal Medicine* 235, no. 2 (1994): 129–35.

83. Ibid., 130.

84. Marcel C. LaFollette, "The Politics of Research Misconduct: Congressional Oversight, Universities, and Science," *Journal of Higher Education* 65, no. 3 (1994): 268.

85. U.S. Department of Health and Human Services, Office of Public Health and Science, *Office of Research Integrity, Annual Report 2001: Office of the Secretary,* 2001. Copy on file with author.

86. Claude Bernard, *An Introduction to the Study of Experimental Medicine,* trans. Henry Copley Green (1865; New York: Schuman, 1949).

87. Robert J. Levine, *Ethics and Regulation of Clinical Research* (New Haven, CT: Yale University Press, 1988), 3.

88. Susan E. Lederer, *Subjected to Science: Human Experimentation in America before the Second World War* (Baltimore: Johns Hopkins Press, 1995).

89. Streptomycin in Tuberculosis Trials Committee, "Streptomycin in Treatment of Pulmonary Tuberculosis," *British Medical Journal* (1948): 769–82.

90. NSABP, "NSABP Timeline."

91. Susan Love is credited with this phrase in Susan Bolotin, "Slash, Burn, and Poison," review of *To Dance with the Devil: The New War on Breast Cancer* by Karen Stabiner (New York: Delacorte, 1997), *New York Times,* April 13, 1997, sec. 7, pg. 8.

92. R. Altman, *Waking Up, Fighting Back,* 161. The papyrus was named for the archaeologist who discovered it.

93. Ibid.

94. A full account of these developments can be found in Barron H. Lerner, "Inventing a Curable Disease: Historical Perspectives on Breast Cancer," in *Breast Cancer: Society Shapes an Epidemic,* ed. A. S. Kasper and S. J. Ferguson (New York: Palgrave, 2000).

95. In fact, Halsted is credited with being the first surgeon to advocate the use of rubber gloves during surgery. Stories about him are legion—it appears that he, too, developed into a larger-than-life scientific figure.

96. William Stewart Halsted, "The Results of Operations for the Cure of Cancer of the Breast from June 1889 to January 1894," *Johns Hopkins Hospital Reports* 4 (1894–1895): 297–350.

97. Marion Yalom, *A History of the Breast* (New York: HarperCollins, 1997), 3.

98. Lerner, "Inventing a Curable Disease."

99. Ellen Leopold, *A Darker Ribbon: Breast Cancer, Women, and Their Doctors in the Twentieth Century* (Boston: Beacon Press, 1999).

100. Quoted in ibid., 67.

101. R. M. Cunningham, "Management of Breast Cancer: Past, Present, Future," *Southern Medical Journal* 69, no. 3 (1976): 260.

102. Fisher et al., "Five-Year Results" and "Eight-Year Results."

103. Richard Saltus, "Reports Back Use of Lumpectomy in Breast Cancer," *Boston Globe,* November 30, 1995, 1.

104. Babette Rosmond wrote under the pseudonym Rosamond Campion. See Campion's *The Invisible Worm: A Woman's Right to Choose an Alternate to Radical Surgery* (New York: Macmillan, 1972), 56.

105. Betty Rollin, *First, You Cry* (New York: Lippincott, 1976); and Audre Lorde, *The Cancer Journals* (San Francisco: Spinsters Ink, 1980).

106. Leslie Hearnshaw, *Cyril Burt: Psychologist* (Ithaca, NY: Cornell University Press, 1979).

107. LaFollette, "Pathology of Research Fraud," 130.

108. William Broad and Nicholas Wade, *Betrayers of the Truth* (New York: Simon and Schuster, 1982).

109. U.S. House of Representatives, Committee on Science and Technology, Subcommittee on Investigations and Oversight, *Fraud in Biomedical Research*, 97th Cong., 1st sess., March 31 and April 1, 1981 (Washington, DC: U.S. Government Printing Office, 1981).

110. Broad and Wade, *Betrayers*.

111. Alexander Kohn, *False Prophets* (New York: Basil Blackwell, 1986).

112. John Dingell's comment to a reporter as reproduced in Daniel Kevles, *The Baltimore Case: A Trial of Politics, Science, and Character* (New York: W. W. Norton, 1988), 15.

113. I say "officially" because I believe institutions still face strong incentives to cover up research misconduct and often succeed in doing so. See Peter Wilmshurst, "The Code of Silence," *Lancet* 349, no. 9051 (1997): 567–69; Lisa B. Keränen, "Assessing the Seriousness of Research Misconduct: Considerations for Sanction Assignment," *Accountability in Research: Policies and Quality Assurance* 13 (2006): 179–205; and Sandra L. Titus, James A. Wells, and Lawrence J. Rhoades, "Commentary: Repairing Research Integrity," *Nature* 453 (2008): 980–82.

114. National Academy of Sciences, "Methods, Definitions, and Basic Assumptions," in R. Bulger, E. Heitman, and S. J. Reiser, eds., *The Ethical Dimensions of the Biological Sciences* (Cambridge, UK: Cambridge University Press, 1993), 107.

CHAPTER 2

1. Denise Grady, "Doctor Doctors Data," *Discover*, January 1995, 104.

2. Ibid.

3. Center for Medical Consumers, Inc., "Can We Trust Clinical Trials? The Falsified Breast Cancer Research," *Health Facts* 19, no. 180 (1994): 1.

4. Dorothy Nelkin, "Science Controversies: The Dynamics of Public Disputes in the United States," in *Handbook of Science and Technology*, ed. Jasanoff et al., 445.

5. Bruno Latour, *Science in Action: How to Follow Scientists and Engineers through Society* (Cambridge, MA: Harvard University Press, 1984), 4.

6. Hyde, *Ethos of Rhetoric*. Hyde develops a Heideggerian sense of ethos that restores an older sense of the term that predates the dominant Aristotelian one. In Hyde's evocative reclamation, *ethos* refers to a common dwelling space, habits learned from being together. This sense of ethos as dwelling place resonates with Chamberlain, "From 'Haunts' to 'Character.'"

7. Gilles Richer, letter to the editor, *NEJM* 330 (1994): 1462.

8. Roger Poisson, letter to the editor, *NEJM* 330 (1994): 1460.

9. Poisson, quoted in Fran Lowry, "Dr. Roger Poisson: 'I Have Learned My Lesson the Hard Way,'" *Canadian Medical Association Journal* 151 (1994): 835.

10. HHS, *Investigation Report: St. Luc*, 2.

11. Unnamed colleague of Roger Poisson, quoted in Alex Robinson, "Science

and Scandal: What Can Be Done about Scientific Misconduct?" *Canadian Medical Association Journal* 151 (1994): 831.

12. Lowry, "Dr. Roger Poisson," 835.

13. Ibid. The question that ends this section is phrased as having been Poisson's sentiment.

14. Loretta M. Kopelman, "Clinical Trials for Breast Cancer and Informed Consent," in *The Voice of Breast Cancer in Medicine and Bioethics*, ed. Mary C. Rawlinson and Shannon Lundeen (Dordrecht, The Netherlands: Springer, 2006), 140.

15. Kathryn M. Taylor, Richard G. Margolese, and Colin L. Soskolne, "Physicians' Reasons for Not Entering Eligible Patients in a Randomized Clinical Trial of Surgery for Breast Cancer," *NEJM* 310 (1984): 1363–67.

16. Ibid.

17. See M. Baum, "Commentary on 'Problems Associated with Randomized Controlled Clinical Trials in Breast Cancer,'" *Journal of Evaluation in Clinical Practice* 4 (1998): 127–28.

18. See, for example, Bernard Fisher, Joseph Costantino, Carol Redmond, Roger Poisson, et al., "A Randomized Clinical Trial Evaluating Tamoxifen in the Treatment of Patients with Node-Negative Breast Cancer Who Have Estrogen-Receptor-Positive Tumors," *NEJM* 320, no. 8 (1989):479–84, where Poisson is listed as fourth coauthor among twenty total authors; and Fisher et al., "Eight-Year Results," where he is third of fifteen authors.

19. Mackenzie Carpenter and Steve Twedt, "Anatomy of a Scandal: Discovering Fraud in Breast Cancer Research a Gradual Process," *Pittsburgh Post-Gazette*, December 26, 1994, A1, A6. I am wholly reliant upon Carpenter and Twedt for this narration of the discovery.

20. Ibid., A1. The B-16 protocol compared chemotherapy and tamoxifen against chemotherapy alone.

21. Ibid.

22. Ibid., A6.

23. HHS, *Investigation Report: St. Luc*, 3.

24. Ibid.; Carpenter and Twedt, "Scandal: Discovering Fraud," A1.

25. Bernard Fisher and Carol Redmond, "Correspondence: Fraud in Breast Cancer Trials," *NEJM* 330 (1994): 1458–60.

26. Ibid., 1458.

27. HHS, *Investigation Report: St. Luc*.

28. Gorman, "Breast Cancer," 52–53.

29. Fisher and Redmond, "Correspondence."

30. Carpenter and Twedt, "Scandal: Discovering Fraud," A6.

31. The other protocols were B-17, B-20-22, and BC-03-4.

32. Carpenter and Twedt, "Scandal: Discovering Fraud," A6.

33. Ibid.

34. Fisher and Redmond, "Correspondence," 1458.

35. Ibid. Readers should recall that OSI became the Office of Research Integrity

(ORI) during the time Poisson was being investigated. In addition, the existence of a "gag order" from talking about the case is disputed.

36. His colleague Dr. R. Guévin initially took over as principal investigator of cancer research for NSABP, followed by Dr. P.-Michel Huet in December 1991. P.-Michel Huet, letter to the editor, *NEJM* 330 (1994): 1462.

37. Ibid.

38. Lawrence K. Altman, "University Is Ordered to Consider Inquiry into Cancer Studies," *New York Times,* April 30, 1994, available at www.nytimes.com/1994/04/30/us/university-is-ordered-to-consider-inquiry-into-cancer-studies.html (accessed July 1, 2009).

39. Roger Poisson, "Opinions," *La Presse,* March 30, 1994, B3.

40. Ibid. *"Mon seul et unique a toujours été de fournir aux femmes chez qui l'on avait diagnostiqué un cancer du sein le meilleur traitement disponible avec le moins de mutilation possible."* All French translations and all errors and awkward phrasings therein are mine, although I much appreciate Jane Elvins's review of my work.

41. Ibid. *"Le cancer du sein, c'est ma profession et ma profession, c'est ma vie!"*

42. Ibid. *"J'ai consacré toute ma vie professionnelle au diagnostic, au traitement du cancer du sein et au suivi des patientes atteintes de cette "maudite maladie". J'ai consacré beaucoup d'énergie et de temps et la grande majorité de mes patientes le savent bien."*

43. Ibid. *"Depuis 1975, j'ai participé à divers protocoles de recherches cliniques dirigés par 'The National Surgical Adjuvant Breast and Bowel Project' (NSABP). J'ai été motivé à faire cela surtout à cause du protocole B-06, une étude américaine qui avait pour but de prouver que la préservation du sein donne d'aussi bons résultats que la mastectomie totale. C'est un sujet qui m'a toujours passionné, surtout depuis la fin des années 60."*

44. Lawrence K. Altman, "The Doctor's World; Flawed Study Raises Questions on U.S. Research," *New York Times,* March 15, 1994, C14, available at www.nytimes.com/1994/03/15/science/the-doctor-s-world-flawed-study-raises-questions-on-us-research.html?pagewanted=1 (accessed July 1, 2009).

45. Ibid.

46. Poisson, "Opinions," B3. *"Je croyais ardemment qu'une patiente qui avait la possibilité de participer à un protocole était très bien traitée et suivie on ne peut mieux. Il me semblait injuste de dire à une femme chez laquelle on avait diagnostiqué un cancer du sein qu'elle n'était pas éligible à recevoir un bon traitement disponible parce qu'elle tombait légèrement à l'extérieur des paramètres du critère 22, particulièrement lorsque ce critère avait peu ou aucune importance intrinsèque oncologique."*

47. Ibid. *"En permettant à ces patientes de participer aux protocoles, je leur donnais accès à de bons soins, certainement aussi bons, si ce n'est meilleurs, que si elles avaient été traitées hors protocol."*

48. Ibid. *"Je n'ai jamais voulu compromettre la santé de mes patientes ou l'intégrité de leurs soins et je ne crois toujours pas que mes patientes en aient souffert."*

49. Both Michael Hyde and I have written about the Hippocratic ethic of medicine. Hyde discusses the relationship between rhetoric and Hippocratic medicine in the context of euthanasia in "Medicine, Rhetoric, and Euthanasia: A Case Study

in the Workings of a Postmodern Discourse," *Quarterly Journal of Speech* 79, no. 2 (1993): 201–24, and *The Call of Conscience: Heidegger and Levinas, Rhetoric and the Euthanasia Debate* (Columbia: University of South Carolina Press, 2001). I critically interrogate medical schools' use of the ideal of Hippocratic medicine in "The Hippocratic Oath as Epideictic Rhetoric: Reanimating Medicine's Past for Its Future," *Journal of Medical Humanities* 21 (2001): 55–68, and I discuss the Hippocratic ethos in "'Cause Someday We All Die': Rhetoric, Agency, and the Case of the 'Patient' Preferences Worksheet," *Quarterly Journal of Speech* 93 (2007): 179–211.

50. For a compelling analysis of how bioethics and courts propelled the autonomy movement, see David Rothman, *Strangers at the Bedside: A History of How Law and Bioethics Transformed Medical Decision Making* (New York: Basic Books, 1991).

51. Paul S. Applebaum, Loren H. Roth, Charles W. Lidz, Paul Benson, and William Winslade, "False Hopes and Best Data: Consent to Research and the Therapeutic Misconception," *Hastings Center Report* 17, no. 2 (1987): 20, 22.

52. Charles Fried, *Medical Experimentation: Personal Integrity and Social Policy* (New York: American Elsevier, 1974).

53. Quoted in Alastair Campbell, Grant Gilbert, and Garth Jones, eds., "The Healing Ethos," in *Practical Medical Ethics* (Oxford: Oxford University Press, 1992), 17.

54. Ibid.

55. L. Altman, "Doctor's World."

56. The terms *research subject* and *research participant* are equally problematic. The first denies agency to those who take part in research, while the latter's egalitarian impulse obscures the power differential implied between researchers and the researched. I use *subject* to highlight this differential.

57. Charles Weijer, "For and Against: Clinical Equipoise and Not the Uncertainty Principle Is the Moral Underpinning of the Randomised Controlled Trial," *British Medical Journal* 321 (2000): 756.

58. Ibid.

59. Ibid.

60. Benjamin Freedman, "Equipoise and the Ethics of Clinical Research," *NEJM* 317 (1987): 144. Freedman's notion of clinical equipoise built on earlier bioethical ideas about the personal care physicians owed to patients, and what he called "theoretical equipoise," when evidence for two treatments was "exactly balanced." See his discussion of theoretical equipoise in "Equipoise," 144. For another take on equipoise, see Fred Gifford, "Freedman's 'Clinical Equipoise' and 'Sliding-Scale All-Dimensions-Considered Equipoise,'" *Journal of Medicine and Philosophy* 25 (2000): 399–426.

61. Freedman, "Equipoise," 144.

62. See R. Levine, *Ethics and Regulation of Clinical Research*, and Freedman, "Equipoise," 144.

63. Freedman, "Equipoise," 144.

64. Ibid.

65. R. Levine, *Ethics and Regulation*, 196.

66. Judith Prestifilippo, Karen Antman, Barbara Berkman, Dwight Kaufman, John Lantos, Walter Lawrence Jr., Robert J. Levine, and Robert J. McKenna, "The Ethical Treatment of Cancer: What Is Right for the Patient?" *Cancer* 72 (1993): S2818.

67. Ibid.

68. Sawyer, "Cancer Researchers' Credibility."

69. Recent debate about the tenability of equipoise may be found in W. Chiong, "Response to Commentators on 'The Real Problem with Equipoise,'" *American Journal of Bioethics* 6, no. 4 (2006): W42–W45, and "The Real Problem with Equipoise," *American Journal of Bioethics* 6, no. 4 (2006): 37–47; H. Mann, "Extensions and Refinements of the Equipoise Concept in International Clinical Research: Would Benjamin Freedman Approve?" *American Journal of Bioethics* 6, no. 4 (2006): 67–69; and F. G. Miller, "Equipoise and the Ethics of Clinical Research Revisited," *American Journal of Bioethics* 6, no. 4 (2006): 59–61. Chiong proposed, inter alia, that clinicians could ease the tension between the therapeutic obligation and equipoise by providing "good enough" care in "Real Problem," 37. Other authors vigorously dissented.

70. Sawyer, "Cancer Researchers' Credibility."

71. "Broke Scientific Rules, Cancer Doctor Admits," *Kitchener-Waterloo (Ontario) Record*, March 31, 1994, A5.

72. Ibid.

73. This point was raised in personal conversation with a legal scholar who did not wish to be named.

74. Cancer researcher Mark C. Lippman made this point in Sawyer, "Cancer Researchers' Credibility."

75. "A Malignant Deception," editorial, *Ottawa Citizen*, March 16, 1994, A8.

76. Barron H. Lerner, "Power, Gender, and Pizzazz: The Early Years of Breast Cancer Activism," in Rawlinson and Lundeen, *Voice of Breast Cancer*, 22.

77. One exception to the privileging of autonomy occurs when, before they become ill, patients have expressed to their health-care providers a clear preference for withholding bad news. In addition, certain cultures and co-cultural groups advocate not sharing with a patient the news that he or she is dying.

78. Thomas L. Beauchamp and James F. Childress make the case for autonomy as the primary bioethical principal in *Principles of Biomedical Ethics*, 5th ed. (New York: Oxford University Press, 2001). While their principalist approach to bioethics has been thoroughly criticized, patient autonomy remains one of the bedrock values of contemporary bioethics. See John Evans, *Playing God? Human Genetic Engineering and the Rationalization of Public Bioethical Debate* (Chicago: University of Chicago Press, 2002), for a critique of principalism.

79. The *Belmont Report* identified respect for persons, beneficence, and justice as ethical principles that should inform biomedical and behavioral research. Na-

tional Commission for the Protection of Human Subjects of Biomedical and Behavioral Research, *The Belmont Report: Ethical Principles and Guidelines for the Protection of Human Subjects of Research* (Washington, DC: U.S. Department of Health, Education, and Welfare, 1979). James F. Childress, Eric M. Meslin, and Harold T. Shapiro have a useful edited collection of essays that outline the past and future of Belmont: *Belmont Revisited: Ethical Principles for Research with Human Subjects* (Washington, DC: Georgetown University Press, 2005). See also Beauchamp and Childress, *Principles.*

80. John Nessa and Kirsti Malterud, "Tell Me What's Wrong with Me: A Discourse Analysis Approach to the Concept of Patient Autonomy," *Journal of Medical Ethics* 24 (1998): 400.

81. Gorman, "Breast Cancer," 52–53.

82. Poisson, "Opinions," B3. "*Les variations en question se rapportaient principalement aux critères d'éligibilité concernant les patientes à se qualifier pour les protocoles du NSABP.*"

83. Ibid. "*Certains sont très importants comme le diagnostic, le stade de la maladie (degré d'envahissement), la qualité de l'acte opératoire, etc.*"

84. Ibid. "*N'ont peu ou pas de valeur oncologique intrinsèque.*"

85. Ibid. "*47% des variations (54 de 115) concernaient le critère établissant le délai maximum de 28 jours entre la date du diagnostic et l'admission dans le protocol.*"

86. Sawyer, "Cancer Researchers' Credibility."

87. L. Altman, "Fall of a Man."

88. Latour, *Science in Action,* 30.

89. Ibid.

90. Gorman, "Breast Cancer," 52–53.

91. L. Altman, "Doctor's World."

92. Barry Came, "'Someone Wants My Skin,'" *Maclean's,* April 11, 1994, 18.

93. "Canadian Doctor Defends Cancer Study Actions," United Press International, March 31, 1994, from http://www.lexisnexis.com (accessed September 13, 2006).

94. Clyde H. Farnsworth, "Doctor Says He Falsified Cancer Data to Help Patients," *New York Times,* April 1, 1994. http://query.nytimes.com/gst/fullpage.html?sec=health&res=9900EED8153FF932A35757C0A962958260 (accessed July 1, 2009).

95. Ibid.

96. Ibid.

97. UPI quotes are from "Canadian Doctor Defends Cancer Study Actions."

98. William Brock, quoted in L. Altman, "Doctor's World."

99. "Doctor Defends Falsifying Data; Claims Critics in U.S. Medical Establishment Out to Get Him," *Montreal Gazette,* March 31, 1993, A3.

100. Farnsworth, "Doctor Says He Falsified."

101. Ibid.

102. "Doctor Defends Falsifying Data."

103. "Canadian Doctor Defends Cancer Study Actions."

104. Farnsworth, "Doctor Says He Falsified."

105. Poisson, *Le Cancer Du Sein S. V. P. Ne Pas Mutiler* (Montreal: Méridien, 1994), 403. "*La public mérite certainement plus de renseignements sur toute cette affaire. J'ai consacré toute ma vie professionnelle au diagnostic, au traitement du cancer du sein et au suivi des patients atteintes de cette 'maudite maladie.' J'y ai consacré beaucoup d'energie et de temps et al grande majorité de mes patients le savent bien.*"

106. Ibid., 418. "*Avec tout ce qu'il offre, ce Monde sera Tien / Et, bien plus encore, tu seras un Homme, mon fils!*"

107. Sawyer, "Cancer Researchers' Credibility."

108. Robinson, "Science and Scandal," 831.

109. Lowry, "Dr. Roger Poisson," 835.

110. Ibid.

111. Ibid.

112. Ibid., 836.

113. Poisson, quoted in Lowry, "Dr. Roger Poisson," 835.

114. Farnsworth, "Doctor Says He Falsified."

115. Ibid.

116. Poisson, letter to the editor, 1460.

117. Poisson, quoted in Kathy A. Fackelmann, "Breast Cancer Research on Trial," *Science News* 145, no. 18 (1994): 282.

118. Poisson, letter to the editor, 1460.

119. "Falsified Cancer Data Merit Strong Measures," editorial, *Vancouver Sun,* March 17, 1994, A18.

120. Randy Allen Harris, "Generative Semantics: Secret Handshakes, Anarchy Notes, and the Implosion of Ethos," *Rhetoric Review* 12 (1993): 127.

121. "Falsified Cancer Data."

122. "Broke Scientific Rules."

123. Jacques Jolivet, quoted in Gorman, "Breast Cancer," 52.

124. L. Altman, "Doctor's World."

125. See Keränen, "Mapping Misconduct," 94–113.

126. Sigal testimony, U.S. House, *Scientific Misconduct,* 29.

127. John Schwartz, "Experts Try to Allay Cancer Fraud Fears," *Washington Post,* March 15, 1994, A3.

128. Gina Kolata, "Breast Cancer Advice Unchanged Despite Flawed Data in Key Study," *New York Times,* March 15, 1994, A1, http://www.nytimes.com/1994/03/15/science/breast-cancer-advice-unchanged-despite-flawed-data-in-key-study.html (accessed July 1, 2009).

129. Michael Zerbe, Amanda J. Young, and Edwin R. Nagelhout, "The Rhetoric of Fraud in Breast Cancer Trials: Manifestations in Medical Journals and the Mass Media—And Missed Opportunities," *Journal of Technical Writing and Communication* 28 (1998): 41.

130. Charisse Jones, "Flawed Cancer Study Haunts Many Women," *New*

York Times March 16, 1994, B7, http://www.nytimes.com/1994/03/16/us/flawed-cancer-study-haunts-many-women.html; and Robin Herman, "Research Fraud Breaks Chain of Trust," *Washington Post,* April 19, 1994, Z6.

131. Farnsworth, "Doctor Says He Falsified."

132. HHS, *Investigation Report: St. Luc.*

133. This point is not meant to suggest that ethics and clinical trial research were not discussed in the 1970s. Indeed, human subjects' research protections were highlighted in the *Belmont Report,* and sporadic public discussion of controversial cases occurred. However, it was not until the late 1980s and early 1990s that there was serious national attention to research misconduct that resulted in changing federal policy.

134. Niels Lynoe, Lars Jacobsson, and E. Lundgren found that researchers held divergent views of what constituted research misconduct. "Fraud, Misconduct, or Normal Science in Medical Research—An Empirical Study of Demarcation," *Journal of Medical Ethics* 25 (1999): 501–07.

135. Charles Weijer, "The Breast Cancer Research Scandal: Addressing the Issues," *Canadian Medical Association Journal* 152 (1995): 1195. *"Les trois raisons invoqueés par le Dr. Roger Poisson pour rationaliser le fait qu'il a utilisé des sujets non admissibles à des essais cliniqiues ne justifient pas la fraude en recherche."*

136. Ibid. *"On peut néanmoins tirer cette affaire certaines leçons sur la conduite des reserches cliniques."*

137. "Doctor Defends Falsifying Data."

138. Ibid.

139. Ware and Linkugel, "Rhetorical Persona," 50.

CHAPTER 3

1. Arthur Levine, "Introduction to Legacy Laureate Bernard Fisher," Address at Medical Grand Rounds, University of Pittsburgh Medical Center, October 27, 2000. I attended this speech.

2. Bernard Fisher, "Insularity with Vision: A Paradigm for Scientific Productivity," Legacy Laureate Address at Medical Grand Rounds, videotape, University of Pittsburgh Medical Center, October 27, 2000.

3. Zagacki and Keith, "Rhetoric, *Topoi,*" 59–78.

4. Center for Medical Consumers, "Can We Trust Clinical Trials?" 1–2.

5. Zeneca Pharmaceuticals, "Heroes Among Us," *Solutions: Business News and Commentary for Zeneca Pharmaceuticals U.S. Employees* 2, no. 3 (1998).

6. See L. Altman, "Fall of a Man."

7. Mackenzie Carpenter, "Fisher's Years of Achievement Crumble Overnight," *Pittsburgh Post-Gazette,* December 26, 1994, A7.

8. Ibid.

9. Ibid.

10. Sources differ on his starting date. For the official version of NSABP history, see the "NSABP Timeline."

11. Fisher, "Insularity with Vision." Fisher later embarked upon several distinct phases of work. He began, for example, what he would later humorously dub his "Promethean Period" when he was "hung up in the sinusoids of the liver," investigating with his brother, Edwin, a 1947 graduate of Pitt's medical school, how a damaged liver could regenerate to its previous size and then cease growing. Soon came his soi-disant Blue Period, in which Fisher, along with Edwin and others, studied hypothermia during the mid- to late 1950s. His coauthored research on the "Effects of Hypothermia upon Induced Bacteremia," "The Effects of Hypothermia of 2 to 24 Hours on Oxygen Consumption and Cardiac Output in the Dog," and "Stressor Effects of Hypothermia in the Rat" conjure images of spanking-white lab coats, caged animals, and gleaming hypodermic needles. In short, Fisher, the boy who used to read books about scientific greats, was embodying the life of a professional research scientist and was well on the way to joining their ranks. See, for example, Fisher, "Insularity with Vision"; Bernard Fisher, F. M. Mateer, C. Russ, and H. Uram, "The Electrolyte Pattern Following Total Hepatectomy," *Surgical Forum of the American College of Surgeons* 4 (1953): 397–401; E. J. Fedor et al., "Effects of Hypothermia upon Induced Bacteremia," *Proceedings for the Society of Experimental Biology and Medicine* 3 (1956): 510–12; B. Fisher, C. Russ, and E. J. Fedor, "Effects of Hypothermia of 2 to 24 Hours on Oxygen Consumption and Cardiac Output in the Dog," *American Journal of Physiology* 3 (1957): 473–76; and E. R. Fisher, E. J. Fedor, and B. Fisher, "Stressor Effects of Hypothermia in the Rat," *American Journal of Physiology* 188 (1957): 470–72. A more robust bibliography of Fisher's publications can be found by entering his name in *Entrez PubMed* (http://www.ncbi.nlm.nih.gov/pubmed), the online search engine of the National Library of Medicine.

12. Bernard Fisher, "Supraradical Cancer Surgery," *American Journal of Surgery* 87 (1954): 155–59; Fisher, "Thoughts from a Journey: Presidential Address before the Twenty-ninth Annual Meeting of the American Society of Clinical Oncology," May 17, 1993, printed in *Journal of Clinical Oncology* 11, no. 12 (1993): 2298. Available at http://tinyurl.com/ph8u4r (accessed September 16, 2009). This statement is echoed in Fisher, "Insularity with Vision."

13. Bernard Fisher, quoted in Leah Kauffman, "Bernard Fisher in Conversation," interview, *Pitt Med* 4, no. 3 (July 2002): 15.

14. Bernard Fisher's recollection of the conversation quoted in ibid.

15. Bernard Fisher, quoted in ibid.

16. Ibid., 15.

17. Fisher, "Thoughts from a Journey," 2298.

18. Ibid.

19. Ibid.

20. NSABP, "NSABP Timeline."

21. Adjuvant therapies accompany other treatments. Fisher, "Thoughts from a Journey," 2298.

22. Carpenter, "Fisher's Years of Achievement."

23. Fisher, "Thoughts from a Journey," 2298.

24. NSABP, "NSABP Timeline."

25. Fisher, "Thoughts from a Journey," 2298.

26. Thomas S. Kuhn, *The Structure of Scientific Revolutions* (Chicago: University of Chicago Press, 1962). See Lerner's discussion of Fisher's Kuhnian rhetoric in Barron H. Lerner, *The Breast Cancer Wars: Hope, Fear, and the Pursuit of a Cure in Twentieth-Century America* (New York: Oxford University Press, 2001): 228–229. For an example of Fisher's revolutionary rhetoric, see Bernard Fisher, "The Revolution in Breast Cancer Surgery: Science or Anecdotalism?" *World Journal of Surgery* 9, no. 5 (1985). Presented in part as the Heath Memorial Award Lecture, M. D. Anderson Hospital and Tumor Institute, November 3, 1982.

27. Lerner, *Breast Cancer Wars*, 139.

28. Ibid., 135. See George Crile Jr., "Breast Cancer: A Patient's Bill of Rights," *Ms. Magazine,* September 1973.

29. Lerner, *Breast Cancer Wars,* 135. It is an important historical note that radiation had taken on increased importance in breast cancer treatment since World War II and was coming to be seen as a therapy that could be used effectively with more limited surgery.

30. Ibid., 135–36.

31. Ibid., 139.

32. Ibid., 138–39.

33. Ibid., 138.

34. Ibid., 139.

35. Ibid.

36. Ibid., 138.

37. Kauffman, "Bernard Fisher in Conversation."

38. Haagenson, quoted in Carpenter, "Fisher's Years of Achievement." Essays appearing in Anne S. Kasper and Susan J. Ferguson, eds., *Breast Cancer: Society Shapes an Epidemic* (New York: Palgrave, 2000), have speculated that the surgical orthodoxy's resistance to Fisher's ideas may have had financial motives, as surgeons would make less money for performing more limited procedures. See also Jane S. Zones, "Profits from Pain: The Political Economy of Breast Cancer," in Kasper and Ferguson, *Breast Cancer,* 119–51.

39. Carpenter, "Fisher's Years of Achievement."

40. Ibid.

41. Don Marquis, "An Argument That All Prerandomized Trials Are Unethical," *Journal of Medicine and Philosophy* 11 (1986): 367–83.

42. Fisher, "Revolution," 656. Some of the quotations used in the middle section of this chapter also appear in Keränen, "Competing Characters."

43. Fisher, "Revolution," 656. The 1993 quotation is from Bernard Fisher and L. Ore, "On the Underutilization of Breast-Conserving Surgery for the Treatment of Breast Cancer," *Annals of Oncology* 4 (1993): 97.

44. Zagacki and Keith, "Rhetoric, *Topoi.*"

45. Fisher, "Revolution," 655; Bernard Fisher, "The Importance of Clinical Trials," *News from the Commission on Cancer of the American College of Surgeons* 2, no. 2 (1991).

46. Fisher, "Revolution," 657.

47. Ibid.

48. Fisher, quoted in Lerner, *Breast Cancer Wars,* 138; Fisher, "Revolution," 655.

49. Kuhn, *Structure of Scientific Revolutions,* 10, 92.

50. Bernard Fisher, "The Evolution of Paradigms for the Management of Breast Cancer: A Personal Perspective," *Cancer Research* 52 (1992): 2371–83.

51. Bernard Fisher, "Justification for Lumpectomy in the Treatment of Breast Cancer: A Commentary on the Underutilization of That Procedure," *Journal of the American Medical Women's Association* 47, no. 5 (1992):169–73. In his similarly worded, coauthored *Annals of Oncology* editorial a year later, he changed the "I" to "we." See Fisher and Ore, "On the Underutilization," 96. Quote from 1970 is in Fisher, "Revolution," 656.

52. Zagacki and Keith, "Rhetoric, *Topoi.*" Lyne and Howe have also examined a revolutionary persona in "Punctuated Equilibria."

53. Unattributed criticism quoted in Lerner, *Breast Cancer Wars,* 139.

54. Fisher, "Insularity with Vision."

55. L. Altman, "Fall of a Man."

56. Steve Twedt, "3 Weeks Shake Cancer Pioneer's 30-Year Record," *Pittsburgh Post-Gazette,* April 3, 1994, A1.

57. Davida Charney, "Lone Geniuses in Popular Science: The Devaluation of Scientific Consensus," *Written Communication* 20 (2003): 215.

58. Center for Medical Consumers, "Can We Trust Clinical Trials?" 1–2.

59. Greenberg, "Dingell and the Breast Cancer Trials," 1089.

60. Ibid.

61. Dr. Thomas Detre and Congressman Sherrod Brown, U.S. House, *Scientific Misconduct,* 166–67.

62. Craig Henderson, quoted in Carpenter and Twedt, "Years of Achievement."

63. Fisher, quoted in Kirsten Boyd Goldberg and Paul Goldberg, eds., "Interim NSABP Leaders Will Not Nominate Chairman, Citing Exec. Committee 'Bias,'" *Cancer Letter* (September 9, 1994): 7.

64. Ibid.

65. Bernard Fisher testimony, U.S. House, *Scientific Misconduct,* 174, 179.

66. Ibid., 174.

67. Carpenter and Twedt, "Scandal: Fisher Describes Ordeal," A1.

68. Kathy Sawyer, "Researcher Accused of 'Lavish Parties'; Dingell Says Pittsburgh Cancer Program Suffered as a Result of 'Garden Spot' Meetings," *Washington Post,* June 16, 1994, A10.

69. Bernard Fisher, quoted in Kirsten Boyd Goldberg and Paul Goldberg, "NCI Apologizes for Mismanagement of NSABP; Says Fisher Resisted Criticism," *Cancer Letter* (April 22, 1994): 11.

70. Ibid.

71. Ibid.

72. Ibid.

73. Ibid., 12.

74. Fisher and Redmond, "Correspondence."

75. Mackenzie Carpenter, "Scientist Launches Public Offensive; Makes Case Researcher Appeals for Reinstatement, Restating of Projects," *Pittsburgh Post-Gazette,* July 13, 1994, B1.

76. Fisher, quoted in ibid.

77. Bruce Chabner, quoted in L. Altman, "Fall of a Man."

78. Twedt, "3 Weeks Shake."

79. Fisher and Redmond, "Correspondence," 1458. Readers should recall that the Office of Scientific Integrity (OSI) became the Office of Research Integrity (ORI) during the time of Poisson's investigation. The existence and parameters of the gag order are disputed.

80. U.S. House, *Scientific Misconduct.*

81. My account of this scene is based on its report in Carpenter and Twedt, "Scandal: Fisher Describes Ordeal," A1.

82. Joseph Onek, quoted in ibid., A11.

83. See Fisher testimony, U.S. House, *Scientific Misconduct,* 171–72.

84. Ibid., 169.

85. Carpenter and Twedt, "Scandal: Fisher Describes Ordeal," A1.

86. Ibid., A1.

87. Onek, quoted in ibid., A10.

88. Ibid., A1.

89. Ibid.

90. Ibid.

91. Goldberg and Goldberg, "NCI Apologizes," 1.

92. Ibid., 2.

93. John Dingell, quoted in ibid., 3.

94. Ibid., 1.

95. "Univ. of Pittsburgh Distances Itself from Fisher" and "NSABP's Pink Sheet: Fisher's Control Had a Downside" are subsections of the larger Goldberg and Goldberg article "Fisher Unable to Answer."

96. Goldberg and Goldberg, "Fisher Unable to Answer," 1.

97. Carpenter and Twedt, "Scandal: Fisher Feared Dingell Inquiry," A11.

98. G. Goldberg, *Enough Already!* 147.

99. See L. Altman, "Fall of a Man," on perceptions of Fisher's arrogance.

100. Fisher testimony, U.S. House, *Scientific Misconduct,* 169.

101. Ibid.

102. Ibid., 170.

103. Ibid.

104. Ibid.

105. Quoted in Fackelmann, "Breast Cancer Research," 286.

106. Ibid.

107. Richard Peto et al., "The Trials of Dr. Bernard Fisher: A European Perspective on an American Episode," *Controlled Clinical Trials* 18 (1997): 7.

108. L. Altman, "Fall of a Man."

109. Fisher, "Thoughts from a Journey," 2298.

110. Ibid.

111. Ibid.

112. Ibid., 2304.

113. Ibid., 2305.

114. Ibid., 2300.

115. Ibid.

116. Ibid.

117. Ibid., 2305.

118. See Carpenter and Twedt's four-part series "Anatomy of a Scandal" and L. Altman, "Fall of a Man."

119. Fisher, "Thoughts from a Journey," 2305.

120. Ibid., 2305.

121. Ibid., 2300.

122. Ibid.

123. Ibid., 2300–01.

124. Drummond Rennie, "Breast Cancer: How to Mishandle Misconduct," *Journal of the American Medical Association* 271 (1994): 1207.

125. Fisher, "Insularity with Vision."

126. Ibid.

127. Ibid.

128. Twedt, "3 Weeks Shake."

129. Ruth Sorelle, "Fisher Defends Study Results at Conference," *Pittsburgh Post-Gazette,* May 17, 1994, A2.

130. However, according to Sorelle, the audience seems to have been divided. Dr. George Peters of Baylor-Sammons Cancer Center in Dallas also received loud applause when he demanded Fisher resign until the ORI's investigation was complete.

131. Sorelle, "Fisher Defends Study."

132. "Taking Advantage: The Completion Begins for Pitt's Prestigious Cancer Study," editorial, *Pittsburgh Post-Gazette,* May 20, 1994, C2.

133. Ibid.

134. Kauffman, "Bernard Fisher in Conversation," 14.

135. The quotations in this paragraph come from ibid., pp. 14, 12, 15, 15, 12, and 14, respectively.

136. Ibid., 13 and 15.

137. Carpenter, "Fisher's Years of Achievement."

138. "A Doctor's Ordeal; Fisher Is a Victim of More Than His Own Misjudgments," editorial, December 29, 1994, D2.

139. Ibid.

140. Ibid.

141. Carpenter, "Scientist Launches Public Offensive."

142. Ibid.

143. Fisher, quoted in ibid.

144. Ibid.

145. These teasers appeared on page 1 of the July 15, 1994, *Cancer Letter*. The article to which they refer, which begins on page 3, is Kirsten Boyd Goldberg and Paul Goldberg, eds., "Fisher Sues Pitt; Demands Reinstatement, Due Process," *Cancer Letter* (July 15, 1994).

146. Kirsten Boyd Goldberg and Paul Goldberg, eds., "Pitt Inquiry Panel Proceedings Suspended; ORI to Take Over NSABP Investigation," *Cancer Letter* (July 22, 1994): 1–4; "NSABP Executive Committee Is Seeking Applications from Surgeons to Lead Group," *Cancer Letter* (July 29, 1994): 1; "ORI Takes Over Misconduct Inquiry of NSABP Officials," *Cancer Letter* (July 28, 1994): 8.

147. These teasers appeared on page 1 of the August 5 and 12 *Cancer Letters*: Kirsten Boyd Goldberg and Paul Goldberg, eds., "Fisher, NSABP Executive Committee File Injunction Seeking Herberman's Removal," *Cancer Letter* (August 12, 1994): 1; "Court Filing by Fisher, Board, Attacks Interim NSABP Leadership," *Cancer Letter* (August 12, 1994): 4; "NSABP Executive Committee Joins Fisher in Suit against Pitt," *Cancer Letter* (August 5, 1994): 1, 8.

148. Fisher, quoted in Goldberg and Goldberg, "Fisher Sues Pitt," 3.

149. Fisher, quoted in Goldberg and Goldberg, "Interim NSABP Leaders," 1.

150. Bernard Fisher, "Breast Cancer Findings Remain Unshaken by Tempest in a Teapot," *Pittsburgh Post-Gazette*, letter to the editor, December 8, 1994, A24.

151. Ibid.

152. Ibid.

153. Fisher, quoted in Goldberg and Goldberg, "Interim NSABP Leaders," 1.

154. Ibid.

155. "Suing for Justice," editorial, *Pittsburgh Post-Gazette*, July 22, 1994, B2.

156. Goldberg and Goldberg, "Fisher Unable to Answer," 1.

157. Barbara A. Seltman, "Justice for Dr. Fisher," editorial, *Pittsburgh Post-Gazette*, January 15, 1994, E3.

158. Ibid.

159. Peto et al., "Trials," 6.

160. "Doctor's Ordeal."

161. Ibid.

162. Ibid.

163. Albert Smolover, editorial, *Pittsburgh Post-Gazette*, May 29, 1994, D2.

164. Mary Ann King, "As a Patient of Dr. Bernard Fisher, I Never Doubted His Integrity," *Pittsburgh Post-Gazette*, September 10, 1994, A16.

165. Ibid.

166. Goldberg and Goldberg, "Second Irregularity," 4.

167. Lewis Kuller, quoted in Carpenter and Twedt, "Scandal: Fisher Feared Dingell," A11.

168. Samuel Hellman, quoted in L. Altman, "Fall of a Man."

169. Susan Love, quoted in Stolberg, "Feeling Betrayed by Science," A1, A22.

170. Ibid., A1.

171. Fisher, "Thoughts from a Journey," 2304.

172. Kauffman, "Bernard Fisher in Conversation," 15. Bracketed text in the original.

173. Fisher testimony, U.S. House, *Scientific Misconduct*, 169.

174. Fisher, quoted in Goldberg and Goldberg, "Second Irregularity," 4.

175. Ibid.

176. Mackenzie Carpenter and Steve Twedt, "Anatomy of a Scandal: Fisher Affair Clouds Future Study," *Pittsburgh Post-Gazette*, December 29, 1994, A1.

177. Ibid.

178. Carpenter, "Scientist Launches Public Offensive."

179. Fisher, quoted in ibid.

180. Sorelle, "Fisher Defends Study."

181. Goldberg and Goldberg, "Second Irregularity," 4.

182. These headlines appear in the June 24 *Cancer Letter*.

183. "Doctor's Ordeal."

184. Anonymous researcher, quoted in Weiss, "NIH: Price of Neglect," 510.

185. Walter Lawrence Jr., quoted in Twedt, "3 Weeks Shake."

186. Ibid.

187. "Doctor's Ordeal."

188. Peto et al., "Trials," 10.

189. Steve Twedt, "End of Dingell Probes a Good Thing, Some Say," *Pittsburgh Post-Gazette*, December 28, 1994, A10.

190. "Bernard Fisher Settles Lawsuit with University of Pittsburgh and Federal Government; Pitt Apologizes for Harm Created," August 28, 1997, copy on file with author.

191. Ibid.

192. See, e.g., Carpenter and Twedt, "Scandal: Fisher Feared Dingell," and Twedt, "End of Dingell Probes."

193. Marylynne Pitz, "Pitt Ordered to Release Documents on Fisher," *Pittsburgh Post-Gazette*, July 12, 1996, C6.

194. Fisher, "Insularity with Vision."

195. Ibid.

196. The microscope under a bell jar was both literal and metaphorical. Fisher stated, "It is evident that the greatest good that can come from a microscope is only when it is focused and the better the focus, the more things that can be seen, and to accomplish this, to keep it in good condition, requires insularity. And that's my paradigm for productivity with evidence." Fisher, "Insularity with Vision."

197. Edward P. J. Corbett, "Foreword," in Ryan, *Oratorical Encounters*, xi.

CHAPTER 4

1. U.S. House, *Scientific Misconduct*, 1.

2. Greenberg, "Dingell and the Breast Cancer Trials," 1089.

3. Sigal testimony, U.S. House, *Scientific Misconduct,* 29.

4. Visco testimony, U.S. House, *Scientific Misconduct,* 13.

5. That so many women were both patients and activists complicates my analysis, because it makes it difficult to characterize the rhetoric of these particular categories. Many representatives of advocacy groups pushed for broader reforms, which would have afforded women more participation in all levels of breast cancer research, but not all did so.

6. Schroder statement, U.S. House, *Scientific Misconduct,* 10.

7. Joseph Gusfield, *The Culture of Public Problems: Drinking-Driving and the Symbolic Order* (Chicago: University of Chicago Press, 1984).

8. Linda Alcoff, "The Problem of Speaking for Others," *Cultural Critique* (Winter 1991–92): 15. Available at http://www.alcoff.com/content/speaothers.html (accessed July 1, 2009).

9. Ibid.

10. C. Miller and Halloran, "Reading Darwin, Reading Nature," 121.

11. American Cancer Society, "ACS History," http://www.cancer.org/docroot/AA/content/AA_1_4_ACS_History.asp? (accessed July 1, 2009).

12. See William Anderson, "We Can Do It: A Study of the Women's Field Army Public Relations Effort," *Public Relations Review* 30, no. 2 (2004): 190.

13. American Cancer Society, "ACS History."

14. Ulrike Boehmer, *The Personal and the Political: Women's Activism in Response to the Breast Cancer and AIDS Epidemics* (Albany, NY: SUNY Press, 2000).

15. Of course, breast cancer was probably discussed in everyday life more than standard histories suggest.

16. "Breast Cancer: Fear and Facts," *Time,* November 4, 1974, http://www.time.com/time/magazine/article/0,9171,945077,00.html (accessed July 1, 2009).

17. Boehmer, *Personal and the Political,* 10.

18. Lerner, "Power, Gender, and Pizzazz," 22.

19. Theresa Montini and Sheryl Ruzek, "Overturning Orthodoxy: The Emergence of Breast Cancer Treatment Policy," *Research in the Sociology of Health Care* 8 (1989): 15.

20. Campion (Rosmond), *Invisible Worm,* 56.

21. See chapter 1, note 105, of the present text.

22. Lorde, *Cancer Journals,* 20.

23. Susan Sherwin, "Personalizing the Political: Negotiating Feminist, Medical, Scientific, and Commercial Discourses Surrounding Breast Cancer," in Rawlinson and Lundeen, *Voice of Breast Cancer,* 6.

24. Rose Kushner, *Breast Cancer: A Personal and Investigative Report* (New York: Harcourt, Brace, and Jovanovich, 1975), 27.

25. Amy Blackstone, "'It's Just about Being Fair': Activism and the Politics of Volunteering in the Breast Cancer Movement," *Gender and Society* 18 (2004): 358.

26. Ibid.

27. Ibid.

28. For a view that situates breast cancer advocacy amid a wider variety of ideological backgrounds and goals, see Maren Klawiter, *The Biopolitics of Breast Cancer: Changing Cultures of Disease and Activism* (Minneapolis: University of Minnesota Press, 2008).

29. Blackstone, "It's Just about Being Fair," 358.

30. L. A. G. Ries et al., eds., SEER Cancer Statistics Review, 1975–2004, National Cancer Institute, Bethesda, MD, http://seer.cancer.gov/csr/1975_2004/, based on November 2006 SEER data submission, posted to the SEER Web site, 2007.

31. Cherise Saywell, "Sexualized Illness: The Newsworthy Body in Media Representations of Breast Cancer," in *Ideologies of Breast Cancer: Feminist Perspectives,* ed. Laura K. Potts (New York: St. Martin's, 2000), 37.

32. Klawiter, *Biopolitics,* xx.

33. Ibid., xxi.

34. Ibid.

35. For Lerner, see chapter 3, note 27, of the present text; Boehmer, chapter 4, note 14; Klawiter, chapter 4, note 28.

36. Barbara Ehrenreich, "Welcome to Cancerland," *Harper's,* November 2001, 45. Ehrenreich offers a smart rejoinder to the "cult of pink kitsch" in sharing her own breast cancer experience. See Phaedra C. Pezzullo, "Resisting 'National Breast Cancer Awareness Month': The Rhetoric of Counterpublics and Their Cultural Performances," *Quarterly Journal of Speech* (2003): 345–65, for a discussion of "pinkwashing" and "greenwashing" as rhetorical strategies.

37. Saywell, "Sexualized Illness," 37.

38. Sherwin, "Personalizing the Political," 8.

39. Alisa Solomon, "The Politics of Breast Cancer," *Camera Obscura: A Journal of Feminism and Film Theory* 28 (1995): 157–77.

40. Harold Varmus, "Testimony of Harold Varmus," U.S. House, *Scientific Misconduct,* 43.

41. Patricia Schroeder, "Statement of Hon. Patricia Schroeder, a Representative in Congress from the State of Colorado," in U.S. House, *Scientific Misconduct,* 9.

42. Jones, "Flawed Cancer Study Haunts."

43. Christopher Anderson, "How Not to Publicize a Misconduct Finding," *Science* 263 (1994): 1679.

44. Crewdson, "Fraud in Breast Cancer Study," A1.

45. Barbara Weber, quoted in Steven Benowitz, "Observers Say Fisher Case Highlights Flaws in System," *Scientist* 11, no. 7 (1997): 7.

46. Jones, "Flawed Cancer Study Haunts."

47. Ibid.

48. Gorman, "Breast Cancer," 52.

49. John Crewdson, "Trust Shaken by Faulty Cancer Study," *Chicago Tribune,* March 27, 1994, A7.

50. Benowitz, "Observers Say Fisher Case Highlights," 7.

51. Ibid.

52. Kolata, "Breast Cancer Advice Unchanged," A1.

53. Crewdson, "Trust Shaken."

54. Herman, "Research Fraud," Z6.

55. Stolberg, "Feeling Betrayed," A1.

56. Ibid, A22.

57. Ibid. Bracketed text in the original.

58. Ibid.

59. Jones, "Flawed Cancer Study Haunts."

60. Twedt, "Study's 'Astonishing' Delay," A10.

61. Ibid.

62. Crewdson, "Trust Shaken."

63. Stabiner, *Dance with the Devil,* 154.

64. Ibid., 154–55.

65. Batt's friend "Caroline" made this remark in Sharon Batt, *Patient No More: The Politics of Breast Cancer* (Charlottetown, P.E.I., Canada: Gynergy, 1994), 357.

66. Ibid.

67. Carolyn Adolph, "Patients Express Alarm about Cancer Research Fraud," *Montreal Gazette,* March 14, 1994, A4.

68. Ibid.

69. Batt, *Patient No More,* 361.

70. Ibid., 362.

71. Ibid.

72. Ibid., 363.

73. André Noel, "Une assemble de patients du docteur Roger Poisson se déroule dans la bisbille," *La Presse,* March 24, 1994, A2, quoted in Batt, *Patient No More,* 374.

74. Batt, *Patient No More,* 363.

75. Ibid., 364.

76. Ibid., 364–65.

77. Ibid., 365.

78. Ibid.

79. Ibid.

80. Ibid., 366.

81. Schroeder statement, U.S. House, *Scientific Misconduct,* 9, 18.

82. Ibid., 10.

83. Sigal testimony, U.S. House, *Scientific Misconduct,* 32.

84. Ibid., 34.

85. Ibid., 30.

86. Saywell, "Sexualized Illness," 40.

87. Ibid.

88. Sigal testimony, U.S. House, *Scientific Misconduct,* 30.

89. Schroeder statement, U.S. House, *Scientific Misconduct,* 9.

90. Herman, "Research Fraud," Z6.

91. Jones, "Flawed Cancer Study Haunts."

92. Ibid.

93. Olympia Snowe, "Statement of the Hon. Olympia Snowe, a Representative in Congress from the State of Maine," in U.S. House, *Scientific Misconduct*, 11.

94. Andrea Rock, "The Breast Cancer Experiment," *Ladies' Home Journal* (February 1995): 145.

95. Ibid.

96. Ibid.

97. Ibid.

98. Ibid., 146.

99. Stabiner, *Dance with the Devil*, 154. See also pages 355–58.

100. Margaret Heuser, "One Incident Shouldn't Hinder Research," *Montreal Gazette*, April 27, 1994, B2.

101. Klawiter, *Biopolitics*, 84. Emphasis in the original.

102. Visco testimony, U.S. House, *Scientific Misconduct*.

103. National Breast Cancer Coalition, "National Breast Cancer Coalition Statement in Response to NSABP Data Falsification," Washington, DC: 1994. Available at http://bcaction.org/index.php?page=newsletter-24q (accessed September 17, 2009).

104. Ibid.

105. Cynthia Pearson, "Testimony of Cynthia Pearson, National Women's Health Network" U.S. House, *Scientific Misconduct*, 23.

106. Ibid.

107. Ibid., 20.

108. Visco testimony, U.S. House, *Scientific Misconduct*, 18.

109. Ibid., 13.

110. Dingell statement, U.S. House, *Scientific Misconduct*, 33.

111. Roush, "John Dingell: Dark Knight," 58.

112. Bernadine Healy, quoted in Carpenter and Twedt, "Scandal: Fisher Feared Dingell," A11.

113. Anonymous researcher, quoted in Rick Weiss, "NIH: Price of Neglect," 510.

114. Unnamed NIH researcher, quoted in ibid., 510.

115. John Dingell, quoted in Bimber and Guston, "Politics by the Same Means," 566.

116. Weiss, "NIH: Price of Neglect," 508.

117. Unnamed health official, quoted in Ford Fessenden, "Calling Science to Account: Hearings on Breast-Cancer Tests," *Newsday*, April 10, 1994, A6.

118. For Kevles, see chapter 1, note 112, in the present text; Crewdson, *Science Fictions: A Scientific Mystery, a Massive Cover-up, and the Dark Legacy of Robert Gallo* (New York: Little, Brown, 2002).

119. Roush, "John Dingell: Dark Knight," 58.

120. Jock Friedly, "Dingell's Investigative Techniques Assailed," *The Hill*, September 3, 2007, 1.

121. Rameshwar Sharma, quoted in ibid.

122. Kirsten Boyd Goldberg and Paul Goldberg, "NCI Audit Verifies Accuracy of Lumpectomy Trial," *Cancer Letter,* October 21, 1994: 1.

123. Friedly, "Dingell's Investigative Techniques," 1.

124. Ibid.

125. However, he has reinvigorated his efforts lately, holding a series of hearings, including ones devoted to biodefense.

126. Varmus and Dingell, U.S. House, *Scientific Misconduct,* 75–76.

127. Friedly, "Dingell's Investigative Techniques," 1. However, there is considerable controversy over the Gallo case and Gallo's innocence, as Crewdson, *Science Fictions,* addresses.

128. Dingell statement, U.S. House, *Scientific Misconduct,* 1.

129. Rebecca Dresser, *When Science Offers Salvation: Patient Advocacy and Research Ethics* (New York: Oxford University Press, 2001), 5.

130. Sonja K. Foss, William J. C. Waters, and Bernard J. Armada, "Toward a Theory of Agentic Orientation: Rhetoric and Agency in *Run Lola Run,*" *Communication Theory* 17 (2007): 206.

131. Lundberg and Gunn, "'Ouija Board,'" 83–106, and Cheryl Geisler, "Teaching the Post-Modern Rhetor: Continuing the Conversation on Rhetorical Agency," *Rhetoric Society Quarterly* 35 (2005): 107–13.

132. For a rehearsal of this position, read Lundberg and Gunn, "'Ouija Board.'"

133. Foss et al., "Toward a Theory," 208.

134. Zillah Eisenstein, *Manmade Breast Cancers* (Ithaca, NY: Cornell University Press, 2001), 101.

135. Foss et al., 207.

136. Concerns about tamoxifen-induced endometrial cancer had been aired before the Datagate scandal broke. Indeed, Congress even held hearings on the matter in 1992. See Jeff Nesmith, "Cancer Death Disclosure Delayed," *Pittsburgh Post-Gazette,* March 3, 1994, A6.

137. Ehrenreich, "Welcome to Cancerland," 48.

138. Pearson, quoted in ibid.

139. Blackstone, "'It's Just about Being Fair,'" 358.

140. Monica Morrow, "Rational Local Therapy for Breast Cancer," editorial, *NEJM* 347 (2002): 1270.

141. Phaedra Pezzullo's "Resisting" includes a discussion of greenwashing.

142. J. Francisca Caron-Flinterman, Jacqueline E. W. Broerse, and Joske F. G. Bunders, "Patient Partnership in Decision-Making in Biomedical Research," *Science, Technology, and Human Values* 32 (2007): 347.

CONCLUSION

1. Adam Marcus, "Fraud Case Rocks Anesthesiology Community; Mass. Researcher Implicated in Falsification of Data, Other Misdeeds," *Anesthesiology News* 35, no. 3 (2009), http://tinyurl.com/kvx4wg (accessed July 2, 2009).

2. Gardiner Harris, "Doctor's Pain Studies Were Fabricated, Hospital Says," *New York Times,* March 10, 2009, online at http://www.nytimes.com/2009/03/11/health/research/11pain.html?partner=rss&emc=rss (accessed July 2, 2009). The "massive" characterization comes from Marcus, "Fraud Case Rocks."

3. In fact, a 2008 survey reported in *Nature* by Titus, Wells, and Rhoades suggested a "sizable disconnect" between observed research misconduct and reports to the U.S. Office of Research Integrity. Extrapolating survey data from 2,212 scientists representing different departments, they noted there could be as many as 2,325 possible misconduct cases a year—a far cry from the 24 misconduct investigations overseen by the ORI each year. Titus, Wells, and Rhoades, "Commentary," 980–82; quotation from page 981. For the story of Bezwoda, see Thomas H. Maugh II and Rosie Mestel, "Key Breast Cancer Study Was a Fraud," *Los Angeles Times,* April 27, 2001, A1.

4. Associated Press, "Scientist Quits after Claims He Faked Data," *New York Times,* June 14, 2003, A13; Benedict A. Carey, "Antidepressant Studies Unpublished," *New York Times* online, January 17, 2008, http://tinyurl.com/r2t9jp (accessed July 2, 2009).

5. Associated Press, "Spectacular Fraud Shakes Stem Cell Field: Scientists Worry South Korean Scandal Will Set Back Legitimate Research," MSNBC, December 23, 2005. Available at http://www.msnbc.msn.com/id/10589085 (accessed July 2, 2009).

6. Norimitsu Onishi, "In a Country That Craved Respect, Stem Cell Scientist Rode a Wave of Korean Pride," *New York Times* online, January 22, 2006, http://www.nytimes.com/2006/01/22/science/22clone.html (accessed July 2, 2009).

7. Ibid.

8. Cultural critic Dave Hickey has advocated that criticism be seen as an act of "writing love songs for people who live in a democracy." At times in this book, my prose has admittedly seemed like anything but a love song. I have criticized some of the words and actions of Drs. Fisher and Poisson; I have expressed concern about the framing of breast cancer patients as knowledge consumers; I have questioned the motivations of federal response to the controversy; and I have taken issue with John Dingell's zeal to stamp out abuse in science. But none of this is meant to detract from the monumental achievements of these people and groups or from the enormous respect I have for each of them. Dr. Poisson has saved lives. Dr. Fisher has profoundly shaped international breast cancer theory and treatment. Congressman Dingell and federal officials have tried to build better oversight mechanisms. Breast cancer advocates have made herculean strides in advancing knowledge and in improving conditions for women with cancer. See Dave Hickey, *Air Guitar: Essays on Art and Democracy* (Los Angeles: Art Issues Press, 1997), 17.

9. Ong, "Voice as a Summons," 92.

10. Lundberg and Gunn, "'Ouija Board,'" 83–106.

11. Shapin, *Scientific Life,* 5.

12. Ibid., 312.

13. Leah Ceccarelli concluded her volume *Shaping Science with Rhetoric* with a discussion of her contributions to four fields. I take my organizational cue from Ceccarelli, even though my audiences differ.

14. Brookey, "Persona," 569–72, and Constantinides, "Duality of Scientific Ethos," 61–72.

15. Craig Waddell, "The Role of *Pathos* in the Decision-Making Process: A Study in the Rhetoric of Science Policy," in R. Harris, *Landmark Essays on Rhetoric of Science: Case Studies*, 145.

16. Lauren Marino, "Speaking for Others," *Macalaster Journal of Philosophy* 14 (2005): 41.

17. Sydney A. Halpern, *Lesser Harms: The Morality of Risk in Medical Research* (Chicago: University of Chicago Press), 17.

18. Aristotle, *Rhetoric*, 1356a.

19. Daniel Sarewitz, "How Science Makes Environmental Controversies Worse," *Environmental Science and Policy* 7 (2004): 397.

20. Taylor, *Defining Science*, 227.

21. Alan Irwin, "Constructing the Scientific Citizen: Science and Democracy in the Biosciences," *Public Understanding of Science* 10 (2001): 1–18; Philip Kitcher, *Science, Truth, and Democracy* (New York: Oxford University Press, 2003); Edna Einsiedel and D. L. Eastlick, "Consensus Conferences as Deliberative Democracy: A Communications Perspective," *Science Communication* 21 (2001): 323–43.

22. See Gordon R. Mitchell and Marcus Paroske, "Fact, Friction, and Political Conviction in Science Policy Controversies," *Social Epistemology* 14, no. 2/3 (2000): 89–108; Irwin, "Constructing the Scientific Citizen"; Kitcher, *Science, Truth, and Democracy*.

23. James Wilsdon, B. Wynne, and J. Stilgoe, *The Public Value of Science; or, How to Ensure That Science Really Matters* (London: Demos, 2005), 19.

24. See Kitcher, *Science, Truth, and Democracy*, and Einsiedel and Eastlick, "Consensus Conferences."

25. Wilsdon et al., *Public Value of Science*, 29.

26. Caron-Flinterman et al., "Patient Partnership," 347.

27. Michael Lynch has identified "elaborate efforts by corporate and political sponsors to create think tanks and even entire fields that mock up the appearance of credibility, objective evidence, and expert authority." Michael Lynch, "Expertise, Skepticism, and Cynicism: Lessons from Science & Technology Studies," *Spontaneous Generations* 1 (2007): 17–25.

28. Peter Sztompa, "Trust in Science: Robert K. Merton's Inspirations," *Journal of Classical Sociology* 7 (2007): 212.

29. John Lyne, "Rhetorics of Inquiry," *Quarterly Journal of Speech* 71, no. 1 (1985): 71.

30. Ibid., 71–72.

31. Charles Percy Snow, *The Two Cultures and a Second Look* (Cambridge, UK: Cambridge University Press, 1964).

Bibliography

Adolph, Carolyn. "Patients Express Alarm about Cancer Research Fraud." *Montreal Gazette,* March 14, 1994, A4.

Alcoff, Linda. "The Problem of Speaking for Others." *Cultural Critique* (Winter 1991–1992): 5–32. http://www.alcoff.com/content/speaothers.html (accessed July 1, 2009).

Alcorn, Marshall W., Jr. "Self-Structure as a Rhetorical Device: Modern Ethos and the Divisiveness of the Self." In Baumlin and Baumlin, *Ethos: New Essays,* 3–36.

Altman, Lawrence K. "The Doctor's World; Flawed Study Raises Questions on U.S. Research." *New York Times,* March 15, 1994, C14. http://www.nytimes.com/1994/03/15/science/the-doctor-s-world-flawed-study-raises-questions-on-us-research.html?pagewanted=1 (accessed July 1, 2009).

———. "Fall of a Man Pivotal in Breast Cancer Research." *New York Times,* April 4, 1994, B10. http://www.nytimes.com/1994/04/04/us/fall-of-a-man-pivotal-in-breast-cancer-research.html (accessed September 25, 2009).

———. "University Is Ordered to Consider Inquiry into Cancer Studies." *New York Times,* April 30, 1994. http://www.nytimes.com/1994/04/30/us/university-is-ordered-to-consider-inquiry-into-cancer-studies.html (accessed July 1, 2009).

Altman, Roberta. *Waking Up, Fighting Back: The Politics of Breast Cancer.* New York: Little, Brown, 1996.

American Cancer Society. "American Cancer Society." http://www.cancer.org.

———. "American Cancer Society History." http://www.cancer.org/docroot/AA/content/AA_1_4_ACS_History.asp (accessed July 1, 2009).

Amossy, Ruth. "Ethos at the Crossroads of Disciplines: Rhetoric, Pragmatics, Sociology." *Poetics Today* 22 (2001): 1–23.

Anderson, Christopher. "How Not to Publicize a Misconduct Finding." *Science* 263 (1994): 1679.

Anderson, William. "We Can Do It: A Study of the Women's Field Army Public Relations Effort." *Public Relations Review* 30, no. 2 (June 2004): 187–96.

Applebaum, Paul S., Loren H. Roth, Charles W. Lidz, Paul Benson, and William Winslade. "False Hopes and Best Data: Consent to Research and the Therapeutic Misconception." *Hastings Center Report* 17, no. 2 (1987): 20–24.

Aristotle. *The Rhetoric and the Poetics of Aristotle.* Translated by W. R. Roberts and I. Bywater. New York: Modern Library, 1984.

Associated Press. "Scientist Quits after Claims He Faked Data." *New York Times,* June 14, 2003, A13.

———. "Spectacular Fraud Shakes Stem Cell Field: Scientists Worry South Korean Scandal Will Set Back Legitimate Research." *MSNBC,* December 23, 2005. http://www.msnbc.msn.com/id/10589085 (accessed July 2, 2009).

Austin, Steve, and Cathy Hitchcock. *Breast Cancer: What You Should Know (But May Not Be Told) about Prevention, Diagnosis, and Treatment.* Rocklin, CA: Prima, 1994.

Batt, Sharon. *Patient No More: The Politics of Breast Cancer.* Charlottetown, P.E.I., Canada: Gynergy, 1994.

Baum, M. "Commentary on 'Problems Associated with Randomized Controlled Clinical Trials in Breast Cancer.'" *Journal of Evaluation in Clinical Practice* 4 (1998): 127–28.

Baumlin, James S., and Tita F. Baumlin, eds. *Ethos: New Essays in Rhetorical and Critical Theory.* Dallas: Southern Methodist University Press, 1994.

Bazerman, Charles. *Shaping Written Knowledge: The Genre and Activity of the Experimental Article in Science.* Madison: University of Wisconsin Press, 1988.

Beauchamp, Thomas L., and James F. Childress. *Principles of Biomedical Ethics,* 5th ed. New York: Oxford University Press, 2001.

Benowitz, Steven. "Observers Say Fisher Case Highlights Flaws in System." *Scientist* 11, no. 7 (1997): 7.

Bernard, Claude. *An Introduction to the Study of Experimental Medicine.* Translated by Henry Copley Green. 1865. Reprint, New York: Schuman, 1949.

"Bernard Fisher Settles Lawsuit with University of Pittsburgh and Federal Government; Pitt Apologizes for Harm Created." August 28, 1997. http://www.asri .edu/bfisher/press_release2.html (accessed September 15, 2002). Copy on file with author.

Biagioli, Mario, ed. *The Science Studies Reader.* New York: Routledge, 1999.

Bimber, Bruce, and David H. Guston. "Politics by the Same Means: Government and Science in the United States." In Jasanoff et al., *Handbook of Science and Technology Studies,* 554–71.

Black, Edwin. "The Second Persona." *Quarterly Journal of Speech* 56 (1970): 109–19.

Blackstone, Amy. "'It's Just about Being Fair': Activism and the Politics of Volunteering in the Breast Cancer Movement." *Gender and Society* 18 (2004): 350–68.

Bloomer, W. Martin. "Schooling in Persona: Imagination and Subordination in Roman Education." *Classical Antiquity* 16, no. 1 (1997): 57–78.

Boehmer, Ulrike. *The Personal and the Political: Women's Activism in Response to the Breast Cancer and AIDS Epidemics.* Albany, NY: SUNY Press, 2000.

Bolotin, Susan, "Slash, Burn, and Poison." Review of *To Dance with the Devil: The New War on Breast Cancer* by Karen Stabiner (New York: Delacorte, 1997). *New York Times,* April 13, 1997, sec. 7, pg. 8.

Bordogna, Francesca. "Scientific Personae in American Psychology: Three Case Studies." *Studies in the History and Philosophy of Biology and the Biomedical Sciences* 36 (2005): 95–134.

Bourdieu, Pierre. *Language and Symbolic Power.* Translated by G. Raymondson and M. Adamson. Cambridge, UK: Polity Press, 1991.

Boyd, Josh. "Public and Technical Interdependence: Regulatory Controversy, Outlaw Discourse, and the Messy Case of Olestra." *Argumentation and Advocacy* 39 (2002): 91–109.

Brante, Thomas. "Reasons for Studying Scientific and Scientific-Based Controversies." In *Controversial Science: From Content to Contention,* edited by Thomas Brante, Steve Fuller, and William Lynch, 177–92. Albany, NY: SUNY Press, 1993.

"Breast Cancer: Fear and Facts." *Time,* November 4, 1974. http://www.time.com/time/magazine/article/0,9171,945077,00.html (accessed July 1, 2009).

"Breast Cancer Study Fraud." *ABC World News Sunday.* Transcript #411, March 13, 1994.

Broad, William, and Nicholas Wade. *Betrayers of the Truth.* New York: Simon and Schuster, 1982.

"Broke Scientific Rules, Cancer Doctor Admits." *Kitchener (Ontario) Record,* March 31, 1994, A5.

Bronowski, Jacob. *Science and Human Values.* New York: Harper and Row, 1965.

Brookey, Robert. "Persona." In *Encyclopedia of Rhetoric,* edited by T. O. Sloane, 569–72. New York: Oxford University Press, 2001.

Brown, Richard Harvey. *Toward a Democratic Science: Scientific Narration and Civic Communication.* New Haven, CT: Yale University Press, 1998.

Brummett, Barry. "The Reported Demise of Epistemic Rhetoric: A Eulogy for Epistemic Rhetoric." *Quarterly Journal of Speech* 76 (1990): 69–72.

Bryant, Donald C. "Rhetoric: Its Functions and Its Scope." *Quarterly Journal of Speech* 39 (1953): 401–24.

Burke, Kenneth. *Counter-Statement.* 1931. Berkeley: University of California Press, 1968.

———. *Language as Symbolic Action.* Berkeley: University of California Press. 1968.

———. *The Rhetoric of Religion: Studies in Logology.* (Berkeley: University of California Press, 1961).

Bush, Vannevar. *Science—The Endless Frontier: A Report to the President.* Washington, DC: U.S. Government Printing Office, 1945.

Came, Barry. "'Someone Wants My Skin.'" *Maclean's,* April 11, 1994, 18.

Campbell, Alastair, Grant Gilbert, and Garth Jones, eds. "The Healing Ethos," *Practical Medical Ethics.* Oxford: Oxford University Press, 1992.

Campbell, Paul Newell. "The Personae of Scientific Discourse." *Quarterly Journal of Speech* 61 (1975): 391–405.

Campion, Rosamond [Babette Rosmond]. *The Invisible Worm: A Woman's Right to Choose an Alternate to Radical Surgery.* New York: Macmillan, 1972.

"Canadian Doctor Defends Cancer Study Actions." United Press International, March 31, 1994. http://www.lexisnexis.com (accessed September 13, 2006).

Carcasson, Martín, and James Arnt Aune. "Klansman on the Court: Justice Hugo Black's 1937 Radio Address." *Quarterly Journal of Speech* 89 (2003): 154–70.

Carey, Benedict A. "Antidepressant Studies Unpublished." *New York Times,* January 17, 2008. http://www.nytimes.com/2008/01/17/health/17depress.html (accessed July 2, 2009).

———. "Criticism of a Gender Theory, and a Scientist under Siege." *New York Times,* August 21, 2007. http://www.nytimes.com/2007/08/21/health/psychology/21gender.html?_r=1& oref=slogin (accessed June 30, 2009).

Caron-Flinterman, J. Francisca, Jacqueline E. W. Broerse, and Joske F. G. Bunders. "Patient Partnership in Decision-Making in Biomedical Research." *Science, Technology, and Human Values* 32 (2007): 339–68.

Carpenter, Mackenzie. "Fisher's Years of Achievement Crumble Overnight." *Pittsburgh Post-Gazette,* December 26, 1994, A7.

———. "Scientist Launches Public Offensive; Makes Case Researcher Appeals for Reinstatement, Restating of Projects." *Pittsburgh Post-Gazette,* July 13, 1994, B1.

Carpenter, Mackenzie, and Steve Twedt. "Anatomy of a Scandal: Discovering Fraud in Breast Cancer Research a Gradual Process." Part 1 of 4. *Pittsburgh Post-Gazette,* December 26, 1994, A1, A6.

———. "Anatomy of a Scandal: Fisher Describes Ordeal as 'Reign of Terror.'" Part 2 of 4. *Pittsburgh Post-Gazette,* December 27, 1994, A1, A6.

———. "Anatomy of a Scandal: Fisher Feared Dingell Inquiry." Part 3 of 4. *Pittsburgh Post-Gazette,* December 28, 1994, A1, A10–12.

———. "Anatomy of a Scandal: Fisher Affair Clouds Future Study." Part 4 of 4. *Pittsburgh Post-Gazette,* December 29, 1994, A1, A10.

Ceccarelli, Leah. *Shaping Science with Rhetoric: The Cases of Dobzhansky, Schrödinger, and Wilson.* Chicago: University of Chicago Press, 2001.

Center for Medical Consumers, Inc. "Can We Trust Clinical Trials? The Falsified Breast Cancer Research." *Health Facts* 19, no. 180 (1994).

Chamberlain, Charles. "From 'Haunts' to 'Character': The Meaning of Ethos and Its Relation to Ethics." *Helios* 11, no. 2 (1984): 97–108.

Charney, Davida. "Lone Geniuses in Popular Science: The Devaluation of Scientific Consensus." *Written Communication* 20 (2003): 215–41.

Cherry, Roger. "Ethos Versus Persona." *Written Communication* 5 (1988): 251–76.

———. "Ethos Versus Persona: Self-Representation in Written Discourse." *Written Communication* 15 (1998): 384–410.

Childress, James F., Eric M. Meslin, and Harold T. Shapiro, eds. *Belmont Revisited: Ethical Principles for Research with Human Subjects.* Washington, DC: Georgetown University Press, 2005.

Chiong, Winston. "The Real Problem with Equipoise." *American Journal of Bioethics* 6, no. 4 (2006): 37–47.

———. "Response to Commentators on 'The Real Problem with Equipoise.'" *American Journal of Bioethics* 6, no. 4 (2006): W42–W45.

Condit, Celeste. "Contributions of the Rhetorical Perspective to the Social Placement of Medical Genetics." *Communication Studies* 46 (1995): 118–29.

Constantinides, Helen. "The Duality of Scientific Ethos: Deep and Surface Structures." *Quarterly Journal of Speech* 87, no. 1 (2001): 61–72.

Corbett, Edward P. J. "Foreword." In Ryan, *Oratorical Encounters,* ix–xi.

Corder, Jim W. "Hunting for Ethos Where They Say It Can't Be Found." *Rhetoric Review* 7 (1989): 299–316.

Cozzens, Susan E., and Edward J. Woodhouse. "Science, Government, and the Politics of Knowledge." In Jasanoff et al., *Handbook of Science and Technology Studies,* 533–53.

Crewdson, John. "Fraud in Breast Cancer Study: Doctor Lied on Data for Decade." *Chicago Tribune,* March 13, 1994, A1, A16.

———. *Science Fictions: A Scientific Mystery, a Massive Cover-up, and the Dark Legacy of Robert Gallo.* New York: Little, Brown, 2002.

———. "Trust Shaken by Faulty Cancer Study." *Chicago Tribune,* March 27, 1994, A7.

Crile, George, Jr. "Breast Cancer: A Patient's Bill of Rights." *Ms. Magazine,* September 1973.

Cunningham, R. M. "Management of Breast Cancer: Past, Present, Future." *Southern Medical Journal* 69, no. 3 (1976): 260–65.

Dingell, John. Statement. U.S. House, *Scientific Misconduct.*

Djerassi, Carl. *Cantor's Dilemma.* New York: Penguin, 1989.

"Doctor Defends Falsifying Data; Claims Critics in U.S. Medical Establishment Out to Get Him." *Montreal Gazette,* March 31, 1993, A3.

"A Doctor's Ordeal; Fisher Is a Victim of More Than His Own Misjudgments." Editorial. *Pittsburgh Post-Gazette,* December 30, 1994, D2.

Dresser, Rebecca. *When Science Offers Salvation: Patient Advocacy and Research Ethics.* New York: Oxford University Press, 2001.

Dunham, Will. "Health Researchers Cleared of Vaccine Misconduct." *Reuter's News,* September 28, 2007. http://www.reuters.com/article/domesticNews/idUSN2845456620070928 (accessed July 2, 2009).

Ehrenreich, Barbara. "Welcome to Cancerland." *Harper's,* November 2001, 43–53.

Einsiedel, Edna, and D. L. Eastlick. "Consensus Conferences as Deliberative Democracy: A Communications Perspective." *Science Communication* 21 (2001): 323–43.

Eisenstein, Zillah. *Manmade Breast Cancers.* Ithaca, NY: Cornell University Press, 2001.

Elbow, Peter. "Introduction: About Voice and Writing." In *Landmark Essays on Voice and Writing,* edited by Peter Elbow. Mahwah, NJ: Hermagoras Press, 1994. xi–xxxix.

Elliott, R. C. *The Literary Persona.* Chicago: University of Chicago Press, 1982.

Ettema, James S., and Theodore L. Glasser. "Narrative Form and Moral Force: The Realization of Innocence and Guilt through Investigative Journalism." *Jour-*

nal of Communication 38, no. 3 (1988): 8–26. Reprinted in *Methods of Rhetorical Criticism: A Twentieth-Century Perspective,* 3rd ed., edited by Bernard L. Brock, Robert L. Scott, and James W. Chesebro, 256–71. Detroit: Wayne State University Press, 1989.

Evans, John. *Playing God? Human Genetic Engineering and the Rationalization of Public Bioethical Debate.* Chicago: University of Chicago Press, 2002.

Ezrahi, Yaron. "The Political Resources of American Science." *Science Studies* 1, no. 2 (1971): 117–33.

Fackelmann, Kathy A. "Breast Cancer Research on Trial." *Science News* 145, no. 18 (1994): 282–85.

"Falsified Cancer Data Merit Strong Measures." Editorial. *Vancouver Sun,* March 17, 1994, A18.

Farnsworth, Clyde H. "Doctor Says He Falsified Cancer Data to Help Patients." *New York Times,* April 1, 1994. http://query.nytimes.com/gst/fullpage .html?sec=health&res=9900EED8153FF932A35757C0A962958260 (accessed July 1, 2009).

Fedor, E. J., B. Fisher, E. R. Fisher, S. H. Lee, and W. K. Weitzel. "Effects of Hypothermia upon Induced Bacteremia." *Proceedings for the Society of Experimental Biology and Medicine* 3 (1956): 510–12.

Fessenden, Ford. "Calling Science to Account: Hearings on Breast-Cancer Tests." *Newsday,* April 10 1994, A6.

"Findings of Scientific Misconduct." *Federal Register* 58, no. 117 (June 21, 1993): 33831.

Fisher, Bernard. "Breast Cancer Findings Remain Unshaken by Tempest in a Teapot." Letter to the Editor. *Pittsburgh Post-Gazette,* December 8, 1994, A24.

———. "The Evolution of Paradigms for the Management of Breast Cancer: A Personal Perspective," *Cancer Research* 52 (1992): 2371–83.

———. "The Importance of Clinical Trials." *News from the Commission on Cancer of the American College of Surgeons* 2, no. 2 (1991).

———. "Insularity with Vision: A Paradigm for Scientific Productivity." Legacy Laureate Address at Medical Grand Rounds, videotape. University of Pittsburgh Medical Center, October 27, 2000.

———. "Justification for Lumpectomy in the Treatment of Breast Cancer: A Commentary on the Underutilization of That Procedure." *Journal of the American Medical Women's Association* 47, no. 5 (1992):169–73.

———. "The Revolution in Breast Cancer Surgery: Science or Anecdotalism?" *World Journal of Surgery* 9, no. 5 (1985): 655–66.

———. "Supraradical Cancer Surgery." *American Journal of Surgery* 87 (1954): 155–59.

———. "Testimony of Bernard Fisher, Former Chairman, National Surgical Adjuvant Breast and Bowel Project, University Of Pittsburgh." In U.S. House, *Scientific Misconduct.*

———. "Thoughts from a Journey: Presidential Address before the Twenty-ninth Annual Meeting of the American Society of Clinical Oncology." May 17, 1993. Printed in *Journal of Clinical Oncology* 11, no. 12 (1993): 2297–2305.

Fisher, Bernard, and L. Ore, "On the Underutilization of Breast-Conserving Surgery for the Treatment of Breast Cancer." *Annals of Oncology* 4 (1993): 96–98.

Fisher, Bernard, Stewart Anderson, Carol K. Redmond, Norman Wolmark, Lawrence Wickerham, and Walter M. Cronin. "Reanalysis and Results after 12 Years of Follow-up in a Randomized Clinical Trial Comparing Total Mastectomy With Lumpectomy With or Without Irradiation in the Treatment of Breast Cancer." *New England Journal of Medicine* 333 (1995): 1456–61.

Fisher, Bernard, Madeleine Bauer, Richard Margolese, Roger Poisson, Yosef Pilch, Carol Redmond, Edwin Fisher, Norman Wolmark, Melvin Deutsch, Eleanor Montague, Elizabeth Saffer, Lawrence Wickerham, Harvey Lerner, Andrew Glass, Henry Shibata, Peter Deckers, Alfred Ketcham, Robert Oishi, and Ian Russell. "Five-Year Results of a Randomized Clinical Trial Comparing Total Mastectomy with or Without Radiation in the Treatment of Breast Cancer." *New England Journal of Medicine* 312, no. 11 (1985): 665–73.

Fisher, Bernard, Joseph Costantino, Carol Redmond, Roger Poisson, David Bowman, Jean Couture, Nikolay V. Dimitrov, et al. "A Randomized Clinical Trial Evaluating Tamoxifen in the Treatment of Patients with Node-Negative Breast Cancer Who Have Estrogen-Receptor-Positive Tumors." *New England Journal of Medicine* 320, no. 8 (1989): 479–84.

Fisher, Bernard, F. M. Mateer, C. Russ, and H. Uram. "The Electrolyte Pattern Following Total Hepatectomy." *Surgical Forum of the American College of Surgeons* 4 (1953): 397–401.

Fisher, Bernard, and Carol Redmond. "Correspondence: Fraud in Breast Cancer Trials." *New England Journal of Medicine* 330, no. 20 (1994): 1458–62.

Fisher, Bernard, Carol Redmond, Roger Poisson, Richard Margolese, Norman Wolmark, D. Lawrence Wickerham, Edwin Fisher, et al. "Eight-Year Results of a Randomized Clinical Trial Comparing Total Mastectomy and Lumpectomy With or Without Irradiation in the Treatment of Breast Cancer." *New England Journal of Medicine* 320, no. 13 (1989): 822–28.

Fisher, Bernard, C. Russ, and E. J. Fedor. "Effects of Hypothermia of 2 to 24 Hours on Oxygen Consumption and Cardiac Output in the Dog." *American Journal of Physiology* 188 (1957): 473–76.

Fisher, Edwin R., E. J. Fedor, and B. Fisher. "Stressor Effects of Hypothermia in the Rat." *American Journal of Physiology* 188 (1957): 470–72.

Foss, Sonja K., William J. C. Waters, and Bernard J. Armada. "Toward a Theory of Agentic Orientation: Rhetoric and Agency in *Run Lola Run*." *Communication Theory* 17 (2007): 205–30.

Freedman, Benjamin. "Equipoise and the Ethics of Clinical Research." *New England Journal of Medicine* 317 (1987): 141–45.

Freircich, Emil J. "Bernard Fisher and the NSABP: Controversy Cannot Tarnish a Career That Helped Millions." Letter to the Editor. *Cancer Letter* 20, no. 15 (1994): 8.

Fried, Charles. *Medical Experimentation: Personal Integrity and Social Policy.* New York: American Elsevier, 1974.

Friedley, Jock. "Dingell's Investigative Techniques Assailed." *The Hill,* September 3, 2007, 1.

Garver, Eugene. *Aristotle's Rhetoric: An Art of Character.* Chicago: University of Chicago Press, 1994.

Geisler, Cheryl. "Teaching the Post-Modern Rhetor: Continuing the Conversation on Rhetorical Agency." *Rhetoric Society Quarterly* 35 (2005): 107–13.

Gibson, Walker. *Persona: A Style Study for Readers and Writers.* New York: Random House, 1969.

Gieryn, Thomas F. *Cultural Boundaries of Science: Credibility on the Line.* Chicago: University of Chicago Press, 1999.

Gifford, Fred. "Freedman's 'Clinical Equipoise' and 'Sliding-Scale All-Dimensions-Considered Equipoise.'" *Journal of Medicine and Philosophy* 25 (2000): 399–426.

Goldberg, George. *Enough Already! The Overtreatment of Early Breast Cancer.* Tucson, AZ: Paracelsus Press, 1996.

Goldberg, Kirsten Boyd, and Paul Goldberg, eds. "Court Filing by Fisher, Board, Attacks Interim NSABP Leadership." *Cancer Letter* (August 12, 1994): 4.

———. "Fisher, NSABP Executive Committee File Injunction Seeking Herberman's Removal." *Cancer Letter* (August 12, 1994): 1–4.

———. "Fisher Sues Pitt; Demands Reinstatement, Due Process." *Cancer Letter* (July 15, 1994): 3.

———. "Fisher Unable to Answer Key Questions, Blames NCI at Second Hearing on NSABP." *Cancer Letter* (June 24, 1994): 1.

———. "Interim NSABP Leaders Will Not Nominate Chairman, Citing Exec. Committee 'Bias.'" *Cancer Letter* (September 9, 1994): 1–8.

———. "NCI Apologizes for Mismanagement of NSABP; Says Fisher Resisted Criticism." *Cancer Letter* (April 22, 1994): 1–7.

———. "NCI Audit Verifies Accuracy of Lumpectomy Trial." *Cancer Letter* (October 21, 1994): 1–4.

———. "NSABP Executive Committee Is Seeking Applications from Surgeons to Lead Group." *Cancer Letter* (July 29, 1994): 1.

———. "NSABP Executive Committee Joins Fisher in Suit Against Pitt." *Cancer Letter* (August 5, 1994): 1, 8.

———. "ORI Takes Over Misconduct Inquiry of NSABP Officials." *Cancer Letter* (July 28, 1994): 8.

———. "Pitt Inquiry Panel Proceedings Suspended; ORI to Take Over NSABP Investigation." *Cancer Letter* (July 22, 1994): 1–4.

———. "Second Irregularity in NSABP Data Found; Fisher Takes Leave as Group's Chairman." *Cancer Letter* (April 1, 1994): 1–5.

Goodnight, G. Thomas. "The Personal, Technical, and Public Spheres of Argument: A Speculative Inquiry into the Art of Public Deliberation." *Journal of the American Forensic Association* 18 (1982): 214–27.

Gorman, Christine. "Breast Cancer: A Diagnosis of Deceit." *Time,* March 28, 1994, 52–53. http://www.time.com/time/magazine/article/0,9171,980381,00.html (accessed June 30, 2009).

Grady, Denise. "Doctor Doctors Data." *Discover,* January 1995, 104.

Greenberg, Daniel S. "Dingell and the Breast Cancer Trials." *Lancet* 343, no. 8905 (1994): 1089.

Gross, Alan G. *Starring the Text: The Place of Rhetoric in Science Studies.* Carbondale: Southern Illinois University Press, 2006.

Gusfield, Joseph. *The Culture of Public Problems: Drinking-Driving and the Symbolic Order.* Chicago: University of Chicago Press, 1984.

Halloran, Michael S. "Aristotle's Concept of Ethos; or, If Not His, Somebody Else's." *Rhetoric Review* 1, no. 1 (1982): 58–63.

———. "The Birth of Molecular Biology: An Essay in the Rhetorical Criticism of Scientific Discourse." In Harris, *Landmark Essays,* 39–50.

Halpern, Sydney A. *Lesser Harms: The Morality of Risk in Medical Research.* Chicago: University of Chicago Press, 2006.

Halsted, William Stewart. "The Results of Operations for the Cure of Cancer of the Breast from June 1889 to January 1894." *Johns Hopkins Hospital Reports* 4 (1894–95): 297–350.

Hardwig, John. "The Role of Trust in Knowledge." *Journal of Philosophy* 88 (1991): 693–708.

Harris, Gardiner. "Doctor's Pain Studies Were Fabricated, Hospital Says." *New York Times,* March 10, 2009, http://www.nytimes.com/2009/03/11/health/research/11pain.html?partner=rss&emc=rss (accessed July 2, 2009).

Harris, Randy Allen. "Generative Semantics: Secret Handshakes, Anarchy Notes, and the Implosion of Ethos." *Rhetoric Review* 12 (1993): 125–60.

———, ed. *Landmark Essays on Rhetoric of Science: Case Studies.* Landmark Essays Series, vol. 11. Mahwah, NJ: Lawrence Erlbaum, 1997.

Hearnshaw, Leslie. *Cyril Burt: Psychologist.* Ithaca, NY: Cornell University Press, 1979.

Herman, Robin. "Research Fraud Breaks Chain of Trust." *Washington Post,* April 19, 1994, Z6.

Hess, David. *Science Studies: An Advanced Introduction.* New York: NYU Press, 1997.

Heuser, Margaret. "One Incident Shouldn't Hinder Research." *Montreal Gazette,* April 27, 1994, B2.

Hickey, Dave. *Air Guitar: Essays on Art and Democracy.* Los Angeles: Art Issues Press, 1997.

Hilgartner, Stephen. *Science on Stage: Expert Advice as Public Drama.* Stanford, CA: Stanford University Press, 2000.

Hotz, Robert Lee. "Most Science Studies Appear to Be Tainted by Sloppy Analysis." *Wall Street Journal,* September 14, 2007, B1.

Huet, P.-Michel. Letter to the Editor. *New England Journal of Medicine* 330 (1994): 1462.

Hyde, Michael J. *The Call of Conscience: Heidegger and Levinas, Rhetoric and the Euthanasia Debate.* Columbia: University of South Carolina Press, 2001.

———. "Medicine, Rhetoric, and Euthanasia: A Case Study in the Workings of a Postmodern Discourse." *Quarterly Journal of Speech.* 79, no. 2 (1993): 201–24.

——. "Rhetorically, We Dwell." In Hyde, *Ethos of Rhetoric*, xiii-xxiv.

——, ed. *The Ethos of Rhetoric*. Columbia: University of South Carolina Press, 2004.

Irwin, Alan. "Constructing the Scientific Citizen: Science and Democracy in the Biosciences." *Public Understanding of Science* 10 (2001): 1–18.

Isocrates. *Antidosis*. Translated by George Norlin. Loeb Classical Library. Cambridge, MA: Harvard University Press, 1982.

Jasanoff, Sheila. "Contested Boundaries in Policy-Relevant Science." *Social Studies of Science* 17 (1987): 195–230.

Jasanoff, Sheila, Gerald E. Markle, James C. Peterson, and Trevor J. Pinch, eds. *Handbook of Science and Technology Studies*. Thousand Oaks, CA: Sage, 1995.

Johnson, Nan. "Ethos." In *Encyclopedia of Rhetoric and Composition: Communication from Ancient Times to the Information Age*, edited by Thersa Enos, 243–45. New York: Garland, 1996.

Jones, Charisse. "Flawed Cancer Study Haunts Many Women." *New York Times*, March 16, 1994, B7.

Kasper, Anne S., and Susan J. Ferguson, eds. *Breast Cancer: Society Shapes an Epidemic*. New York: Palgrave, 2000.

Kauffman, Leah. "Bernard Fisher in Conversation." Interview. *Pitt Med* 4, no. 3 (July 2002): 12–15. http://pittmed.health.pitt.edu/JUL_2002/feature_BFisher .pdf (accessed July 1, 2009).

Keränen, Lisa. "Assessing the Seriousness of Research Misconduct: Considerations for Sanction Assignment." *Accountability in Research: Policies and Quality Assurance* 13 (2006): 179–205.

——. "'Cause Someday We All Die': Rhetoric, Agency, and the Case of the 'Patient' Preferences Worksheet." *Quarterly Journal of Speech* 93 (2007) 179–211.

——. "Competing Characters in Science-Based Controversy: A Framework for Analysis," In *Understanding Science: New Agendas for Communication*, edited by LeeAnn Kahlor and Patricia Stout. New York: Routledge, 2010. 133–60.

——. "The Hippocratic Oath as Epideictic Rhetoric: Reanimating Medicine's Past for Its Future." *Journal of Medical Humanities* 21 (2001): 55–68.

——. "Mapping Misconduct: Demarcating Legitimate Science from 'Fraud' in the B-06 Lumpectomy Study." *Argumentation and Advocacy* (2005): 94–113.

Kevles, Daniel J. *The Baltimore Case: A Trial of Politics, Science, and Character*. New York: W. W. Norton, 1988.

King, Mary Ann. "As a Patient of Dr. Bernard Fisher, I Never Doubted His Integrity." Letter to the Editor. *Pittsburgh Post-Gazette*, September 10, 1994, A16.

Kitcher, Philip. *Science, Truth, and Democracy*. New York: Oxford University Press, 2003.

Klawiter, Maren. *The Biopolitics of Breast Cancer: Changing Cultures of Disease and Activism*. Minneapolis: University of Minnesota Press, 2008.

Kohn, Alexander. *False Prophets*. New York: Basil Blackwell, 1986.

Kolata, Gina. "Breast Cancer Advice Unchanged Despite Flawed Data in Key

Study." *New York Times,* March 15, 1994, section A1. http://www.nytimes.com/ 1994/03/15/science/breast-cancer-advice-unchanged-despite-flawed-data-in-key-study.html (accessed July 1, 2009).

Kopelman, Loretta M. "Clinical Trials for Breast Cancer and Informed Consent." In Rawlinson and Lundeen, *Voice of Breast Cancer,* 133–61.

Kuhn, Thomas S. *The Structure of Scientific Revolutions.* Chicago: University of Chicago Press, 1962.

Kushner, Rose. *Breast Cancer: A Personal and Investigative Report.* New York: Harcourt, Brace, and Jovanovich, 1975.

LaFollette, Marcel C. "The Pathology of Research Fraud: The History and Politics of the US Experience." *Journal of Internal Medicine* 235 (1994): 129–35.

———. "The Politics of Research Misconduct: Congressional Oversight, Universities, and Science." *Journal of Higher Education* 65, no. 3 (1994): 261–87.

Latour, Bruno. *Science in Action: How to Follow Scientists and Engineers Through Society.* Cambridge, MA: Harvard University Press, 1984.

Lederer, Susan E. *Subjected to Science: Human Experimentation in America before the Second World War.* Baltimore: Johns Hopkins University Press, 1995.

Leopold, Ellen. *A Darker Ribbon: Breast Cancer, Women, and Their Doctors in the Twentieth Century.* Boston: Beacon Press, 1999.

Lerner, Barron H. *The Breast Cancer Wars: Hope, Fear, and the Pursuit of a Cure in Twentieth-Century America.* New York: Oxford University Press, 2001.

———. "Inventing a Curable Disease: Historical Perspectives on Breast Cancer." In *Breast Cancer: Society Shapes An Epidemic,* edited by A. S. Kasper and S. J. Ferguson. New York: Palgrave, 2000.

———. "Power, Gender, and Pizzazz: The Early Years of Breast Cancer Activism." In Rawlinson and Lundeen, *Voice of Breast Cancer,* 21–30.

Lessl, Tom. "The Priestly Voice." *Quarterly Journal of Speech* 75 (1989): 183–97.

Levine, Arthur. "Introduction to Legacy Laureate Bernard Fisher." Address at Medical Grand Rounds. University of Pittsburgh Medical Center, October 27, 2000. Videotape.

Levine, Robert J. *Ethics and Regulation of Clinical Research.* New Haven, CT: Yale University Press, 1988.

Lorde, Audre. *The Cancer Journals.* San Francisco: Spinsters Ink, 1980.

Lowry, Fran. "Dr. Roger Poisson: 'I Have Learned My Lesson the Hard Way.'" *Canadian Medical Association Journal* 151 (1994): 835–37.

Lundberg, Christian, and Joshua Gunn. "'Ouija Board, Are There Any Communications?': Agency, Ontotheology, and the Death of the Humanist Subject; or, Continuing the ARS Conversation." *Rhetoric Society Quarterly* 35 (2005): 83–106.

Lynch, Michael. "Expertise, Skepticism, and Cynicism: Lessons from Science and Technology Studies." *Spontaneous Generations* 1 (2007): 17–25.

Lyne, John. "Rhetorics of Inquiry." *Quarterly Journal of Speech* 71 (1985): 65–73.

Lyne, John, and Henry F. Howe. "'Punctuated Equilibria': Rhetorical Dynamics of Science Controversy." *Quarterly Journal of Speech* 72 (1986): 132–47.

Lynoe, Niels, Lars Jacobsson, and E. Lundgren. "Fraud, Misconduct, or Normal Science in Medical Research—An Empirical Study of Demarcation." *Journal of Medical Ethics* 25 (1999): 501–07.

"A Malignant Deception." Editorial. *Ottawa Citizen,* March 16, 1994, A8.

Mann, H. "Extensions and Refinements of the Equipoise Concept in International Clinical Research: Would Benjamin Freedman Approve?" *American Journal of Bioethics* 6, no. 4 (2006): 67–69.

Marcus, Adam. "Fraud Case Rocks Anesthesiology Community; Mass. Researcher Implicated in Falsification of Data, Other Misdeeds." *Anesthesiology News* 35, no. 3 (2009). http://www.anesthesiologynews.com/index.aspses=ogst&section_id=3&show=dept&article_id=12634 (accessed July 2, 2009).

Marino, Lauren. "Speaking for Others." *Macalaster Journal of Philosophy* 14 (2005): 35–45.

Marquis, Don. "An Argument That All Prerandomized Trials Are Unethical." *Journal of Medicine and Philosophy* 11 (1986): 367–83.

Marshall, Eliot. "Tamoxifen: Hanging in the Balance." *Science* 264, no. 5165 (1994): 1524–27.

Martin, Brian. "Strategies for Dissenting Scientists." *Journal of Scientific Exploration* 12 (1998): 605–16. http://www.uow.edu.au/arts/sts/bmartin/pubs/98jse.html (accessed July 1, 2009).

Maugh II, Thomas H., and Rosie Mestel. "Key Breast Cancer Study Was a Fraud." *Los Angeles Times,* April 27, 2001, A1.

Mauss, Marcel. *Une Catégorie de L'espirit Humain: La Notion de Personne, celle de "Moi".* [A Category of the Human Mind: The Notion of the Person, the Notion of the "Self"]. 1938. Reprint, London: Huxley, 1979.

Merton, Robert K. "The Normative Structure of Science." In Merton, *Sociology of Science,* 254–66.

———. *Sociology of Science: Theoretical and Empirical Investigations,* edited by Norman W. Storer. 1942. Reprint, Chicago: University of Chicago Press, 1979. Originally "A Note on Science and Democracy." *Journal of Legal and Political Sociology* 1 (1942): 115–26.

Miller, Carolyn R. "Technology as a Form of Consciousness: A Study of Contemporary Ethos." *Central States Speech Journal* 29 (1978): 228–36.

Miller, Carolyn R., and S. Michael Halloran. "Reading Darwin, Reading Nature; or, on the Ethos of Historical Science." In *Understanding Scientific Prose,* edited by Jack Selzer, 106–26. Madison: University of Wisconsin Press, 1993.

Miller, F. G. "Equipoise and the Ethics of Clinical Research Revisited." *American Journal of Bioethics* 6, no. 4 (2006): 59–61.

Mitchell, Gordon R. *Strategic Deception: Rhetoric, Science and Politics in Missile Defense Advocacy.* East Lansing: Michigan State University Press, 2000.

Mitchell, Gordon R., and Marcus Paroske. "Fact, Friction, and Political Conviction in Science Policy Controversies." *Social Epistemology* 14, no. 2/3 (2000): 89–108.

Montini, Theresa, and Sheryl Ruzek. "Overturning Orthodoxy: The Emergence of Breast Cancer Treatment Policy." *Research in the Sociology of Health Care* 8 (1989): 3–32.

Morris III, Charles E. "Pink Herring and the Fourth Persona: J. Edgar Hoover's Sex Crime Panic." In *Readings in Rhetorical Criticism,* 3rd ed., edited by Carl Burgchardt, 664–82. State College, PA: Strata, 2005.

Morrow, Monica. "Rational Local Therapy for Breast Cancer." Editorial. *New England Journal of Medicine* 347 (2002): 1270–71.

National Academy of Sciences. "Methods, Definitions, and Basic Assumptions." In *The Ethical Dimensions of the Biological Sciences,* edited by R. Bulger, E. Heitman, and S. J. Reiser, 106–13. 1993. Reprint, Cambridge, UK: Cambridge University Press, 1994.

National Breast Cancer Coalition. "National Breast Cancer Coalition Statement in Response to NSABP Data Falsification." Washington, DC: 1994. http://bcaction.org/index.php?page=newsletter-24q (accessed September 23, 2009).

National Commission for the Protection of Human Subjects of Biomedical and Behavioral Research. *The Belmont Report: Ethical Principles and Guidelines for the Protection of Human Subjects of Research.* Washington, DC: U.S. Department of Health, Education, and Welfare, 1979.

National Institutes of Health. "Treatment of Early-Stage Breast Cancer: *NIH Consensus Statement Online.*" 8, no. 6 (1990): 1–19. http://consensus.nih.gov/1990/1990EarlyStageBreastCancer081html.htm (accessed June 29, 2009).

Nelkin, Dorothy. "Science Controversies: The Dynamics of Public Disputes in the United States." In Jasanoff et al., *Handbook of Science and Technology,* 444–56.

Nesmith, Jeff. "Cancer Death Disclosure Delayed." *Pittsburgh Post-Gazette,* March 3, 1994, A6.

Nessa, John, and Kirsti Malterud. "Tell Me What's Wrong with Me: A Discourse Analysis Approach to the Concept of Patient Autonomy." *Journal of Medical Ethics* 24 (1998): 394–400.

Noel, André. "Une assemble de patients du docteur Roger Poisson se déroule dans la bisbille." *La Presse,* March 24, 1994, A2.

Nothstine, William L., Carole Blair, and Gary A. Copeland, eds. *Critical Questions: Invention, Creativity, and the Criticism of Discourse and Media.* New York: St. Martin's, 1994.

———. "Invention in Media and Rhetorical Criticism: A General Orientation." In Nothstine, Blair, and Copeland, *Critical Questions,* 3–14.

———. "Professionalization and the Eclipse of Critical Invention." In Nothstine, Blair, and Copeland, *Critical Questions,* 15–63.

NSABP. "NSABP Timeline." http://www.nsabp.pitt.edu/NSABP_Timeline.pdf (accessed September 1, 2009).

Ong, Walter J. "Voice as a Summons for Belief." In *The Barbarian Within and Other Fugitive Essays and Studies,* 80–105. New York: Macmillan, 1962.

Onishi, Norimitsu. "In a Country That Craved Respect, Stem Cell Scientist Rode

a Wave of Korean Pride." *New York Times* online, January 22, 2006. http://www
.nytimes.com/2006/01/22/science/22clone.html (accessed July 2, 2009).

Pascal, Chris B. "Misconduct Annotations." *Science* 274, no. 5290 (1996): 1065–69.

Patterson, James T. *The Dread Disease: Cancer and Modern American Culture.* Cambridge, MA: Harvard University Press, 1987.

Pearson, Cynthia. "Testimony of Cynthia Pearson, National Women's Health Network." In U.S. House, *Scientific Misconduct.*

Peto, Richard, Rory Collins, David Sackett, Janet Darbyshire, Abdel Babiker, Marc Buyse, Helen Stewart, et al. "The Trials of Dr. Bernard Fisher: A European Perspective on an American Episode." *Controlled Clinical Trials* 18 (1997): 1–13.

Pezzullo, Phaedra C. "Resisting 'National Breast Cancer Awareness Month': The Rhetoric of Counterpublics and Their Cultural Performances." *Quarterly Journal of Speech* (2003): 345–65.

Pitz, Marylynne. "Pitt Ordered to Release Documents on Fisher." *Pittsburgh Post-Gazette,* July 12, 1996, C6.

Poisson, Roger. *Le Cancer Du Sein S. V. P. Ne Pas Mutiler.* Montreal: Méridien, 1994..

———. Letter to the Editor. *New England Journal of Medicine* 330 (1994): 1460.

———. "Opinions." *La Presse,* March 30, 1994, B3.

Prelli, Lawrence J. *A Rhetoric of Science: Inventing Scientific Discourse.* Columbia: University of South Carolina Press, 1989.

Prestifilippo, Judith, Karen Antman, Barbara Berkman, Dwight Kaufman, John Lantos, Walter Lawrence Jr., Robert J. Levine, and Robert J. McKenna. "The Ethical Treatment of Cancer: What Is Right for the Patient?" *Cancer* 72 (1993): S2816–19.

Rapp, Rayna. "Accounting for Amniocentesis." In *Knowledge, Power, and Practice: The Anthropology of Health,* edited by S. Lindenbaum and M. Lock, 55–76. Berkeley: University of California Press, 1993.

Rawlinson, Mary C., and Shannon Lundeen, eds. *The Voice of Breast Cancer in Medicine and Bioethics.* Dordrecht, The Netherlands: Springer, 2006.

Rennie, Drummond. "Breast Cancer: How to Mishandle Misconduct." *Journal of the American Medical Association* 271, no. 15 (1994): 1205–07.

Richer, Gilles. Letter to the Editor. *New England Journal of Medicine* 330 (1994): 1462.

Ries, L. A. G. et al., eds., "SEER Cancer Statistics Review, 1975–2004, National Cancer Institute." Bethesda, MD. http://seer.cancer.gov/csr/1975_2004/. Based on November 2006 SEER data submission, posted to the SEER Web site, 2007.

Robinson, Alex. "Science and Scandal: What Can Be Done about Scientific Misconduct?" *Canadian Medical Association Journal* 151 (1994): 831–34.

Rock, Andrea. "The Breast Cancer Experiment." *Ladies' Home Journal* (February 1995): 145–51, 220.

Rollin, Betty. *First, You Cry.* New York: Lippincott, 1976.

Rorty, Richard. "Science as Solidarity." In *Objectivity, Relativism, and Truth*, 35–45. New York: Cambridge University Press, 1991.

Rosmond, Babette [Rosamond Campion, pseud.]. *The Invisible Worm: A Woman's Right to Choose an Alternate to Radical Surgery*. New York: Macmillan, 1972.

Roszak, Theodore. *The Making of Counter Culture*. New York: Anchor Books, 1969.

Rothman, David. *Strangers at the Bedside: A History of How Law and Bioethics Transformed Medical Decision Making*. New York, Basic Books, 1991.

Roush, Wade. "John Dingell: Dark Knight of Science." *Technology Review* 95 (January 1992): 56–62.

Runquist, Mark. "The Rhetoric of Geology: Ethos in the Writing of North American Geologists, 1823–1988." *Journal of Technical Writing and Communication* 22, no. 4 (1992): 387–404.

Ryan, Halford Ross. "Kategoria and Apologia: On Their Rhetorical Criticism as a Speech Set." *Quarterly Journal of Speech* 68 (1982): 254–61.

———, ed. *Oratorical Encounters: Selected Studies and Sources of Twentieth-Century Political Accusations and Apologies*. New York: Greenwood Press, 1988.

Saltus, Richard. "Reports Back Use of Lumpectomy in Breast Cancer." *Boston Globe*, November 30, 1995, 1.

Sarewitz, Daniel. "How Science Makes Environmental Controversies Worse." *Environmental Science and Policy* 7 (2004): 385–403.

Sawyer, Kathy. "Cancer Researcher's Credibility Ailing; Exposure of Surgeon's 13-Year Deception Has Heavy Public Impact." *Washington Post*, April 13, 1994, A1.

———. "Researcher Accused of 'Lavish Parties'; Dingell Says Pittsburgh Cancer Program Suffered as a Result of 'Garden Spot' Meetings." *Washington Post*, June 16, 1994, A10.

Saywell, Cherise. "Sexualized Illness: The Newsworthy Body in Media Representations of Breast Cancer." In *Ideologies of Breast Cancer: Feminist Perspectives*, edited by Laura K. Potts, 37–62. New York: St. Martin's, 2000.

Schroeder, Patricia. "Statement of the Hon. Patricia Schroeder, a Representative in Congress from the State of Colorado." In U.S. House, *Scientific Misconduct*.

Schwartz, John. "Experts Try to Allay Cancer Fraud Fears." *Washington Post*, March 15, 1994, A3.

Scott, Robert L. "On Viewing Rhetoric as Epistemic." *Central States Speech Journal* 18 (1967): 9–17.

Segal, Judy Z. *Health and the Rhetoric of Medicine*. Carbondale: Southern Illinois University Press, 2006.

Segal, Judy, and Alan Richardson. "Introduction: Scientific Ethos: Authority, Authorship, and Trust in the Sciences." *Configurations* 11, no. 2 (2003): 137–44.

Seltman, Barbara A. "Justice for Dr. Fisher." Editorial. *Pittsburgh Post-Gazette*, January 15, 1994, E3.

Shapin, Steven. *The Scientific Life: A Moral History of a Late Modern Vocation*. Chicago: University of Chicago Press, 2008.

Sherwin, Susan. "Personalizing the Political: Negotiating Feminist, Medical, Scientific, and Commercial Discourses Surrounding Breast Cancer." In Rawlinson and Lundeen, *The Voice of Breast Cancer in Medicine and Bioethics*, 3–19.

Sigal, Jill Lea. "Testimony of Jill Lea Sigal, Consultant, Washington, DC." In U.S. House, *Scientific Misconduct*.

Simons, Herbert W., ed. *The Rhetorical Turn: Invention and Persuasion in the Conduct of Inquiry*. Chicago: University of Chicago Press, 1990.

Smolover, Albert. "Our City Fathers Should Be Busy Defending Pitt and Fisher." Editorial. *Pittsburgh Post-Gazette*, May 27, 1994, D2.

Snow, Charles Percy. *The Two Cultures and a Second Look*. Cambridge, UK: Cambridge University Press, 1964.

Snowe, Olympia. "Statement of the Hon. Olympia Snowe, a Representative in Congress from the State of Maine." In U.S. House, *Scientific Misconduct*.

Solomon, Alisa. "The Politics of Breast Cancer." *Camera Obscura: A Journal of Feminism and Film Theory* 28 (1995): 157–77.

Sorelle, Ruth. 1994. "Fisher Defends Study Results at Conference." *Pittsburgh-Post-Gazette*, May 17, 1994, A2.

Srikameswaran, Anita. "20-year Study Shows Lumpectomies Work." *Pittsburgh Post-Gazette*, October 17, 2002. www.post-gazette.com/healthscience/20021017breast1017P2.asp (accessed September 23, 2009).

Stabiner, Karen. *To Dance with the Devil: The New War on Breast Cancer: Politics, Power, People*. New York: Delacorte, 1997.

Stolberg, Sheryl. "Feeling Betrayed by Science; A Scandal over Faked Data in a Breast Cancer Study Has Left Patients Reeling and a Pioneering Doctor in Disgrace." *Los Angeles Times*, April 1, 1994, A1, A22.

Streptomycin in Tuberculosis Trials Committee. "Streptomycin in Treatment of Pulmonary Tuberculosis." *British Medical Journal* (1948): 769–82.

"Suing for Justice." Editorial. *Pittsburgh Post-Gazette*, July 22, 1994, B2.

Sztompa, Peter. "Trust in Science: Robert K. Merton's Inspirations." *Journal of Classical Sociology* 7 (2007): 211–20.

"Taking Advantage: The Completion Begins for Pitt's Prestigious Cancer Study." Editorial. *Pittsburgh Post-Gazette*, May 20, 1994, C2.

Taylor, Charles Alan. *Defining Science: A Rhetoric of Demarcation*. Madison: University of Wisconsin Press, 1996.

Taylor, Kathy M., Richard G. Margolese, and Colin L. Soskolne. "Physicians' Reasons for Not Entering Eligible Patients in a Randomized Clinical Trial of Surgery for Breast Cancer." *New England Journal of Medicine* 310 (1984): 1363–67.

Thurs, Daniel Patrick. *Science Talk: Changing Notions of Science in American Popular Culture*. New Brunswick, NJ: Rutgers University Press, 2007.

Titus, Sandra L., James A. Wells, and Lawrence J. Rhoades. "Commentary: Repairing Research Integrity." *Nature* 453 (2008): 980–82.

Turner, Stephen. "Merton's Norms in Political and Intellectual Context." *Journal of Classical Sociology* 7 (2007): 161–78.

Twedt, Steve. "3 Weeks Shake Cancer Pioneer's 30-Year Record." *Pittsburgh Post-Gazette,* April 3, 1994, A1.

———. "Data Problems Cited at 11 Cancer Centers." *Pittsburgh Post-Gazette,* June 16, 1994, A12.

———. "End of Dingell Probes a Good Thing, Some Say." *Pittsburgh Post-Gazette,* December 28, 1994, A10.

———. "Study's 'Astonishing' Delay; Medical Journal Critical of Wait to Reveal Falsified Breast Cancer Data." *Pittsburgh Post-Gazette,* April 20, 1994, A10.

University of Pittsburgh. "Bernard Fisher." *University Times* 30, no. 2, September 11, 1997. http://tinyurl.com/myfxtc (accessed June 30, 2009).

———. "Fisher Drops Suit in Exchange for Apology, $2.75 Million; University Administrators Credited with Bringing about Settlement." *University Times* 30, no. 2, September 11, 1997. http://tinyurl.com/p8l3ca (accessed June 30, 2009).

———. "Public Statement Incidental to Termination of Litigation in RE: Fisher vs. University of Pittsburgh, et al." *University Times* 30, no. 2, September 11, 1997. http://tinyurl.com/lh6upb (accessed June 30, 2009).

U.S. Department of Health and Human Services. Office of Research Integrity. *Investigation Report: St. Luc Hospital NSABP Project.* 1993.

———. Office of Public Health and Science. *Office of Research Integrity, Annual Report 2001: Office of the Secretary.* 2001.

U.S. House of Representatives. Committee on Science and Technology. Subcommittee on Investigations and Oversight. *Fraud in Biomedical Research.* 97th Congress, 1st session, March 31 and April 1, 1981. Washington, DC: U.S. Government Printing Office, 1981.

———. Subcommittee on Oversight and Investigations of the Committee on Energy and Commerce. *Scientific Misconduct in Breast Cancer Research.* 103rd Congress, 2nd session, April 13 and June 15, 1994. Washington, DC: United States Government Printing Office, 1994. Full text available at http://www.archive.org/stream/scientificmiscon00unit/scientificmiscon00unit_djvu.txt (accessed July 1, 2009).

Varmus, Harold. "Testimony of Harold Varmus, Director, National Institutes of Health." In U.S. House, *Scientific Misconduct.*

Visco, Fran. "Testimony of Fran Visco, President, National Breast Cancer Coalition." In U.S. House, *Scientific Misconduct.*

Waddell, Craig. "The Role of *Pathos* in the Decision-Making Process: A Study in the Rhetoric of Science Policy." In Harris, *Landmark Essays,* 127–49.

Wander, Philip. "The Third Persona: An Ideological Turn in Rhetorical Criticism." *Central States Speech Journal* 35 (1984): 197–216.

Ware, B. L., and Wil A. Linkugel. "The Rhetorical Persona: Marcus Garvey as Black Moses." *Communication Monographs* 49 (1982): 50–62.

———. "They Spoke in Defense of Themselves: On the Generic Criticism of *Apologia.*" *Quarterly Journal of Speech* 59 (1973): 273–83.

Watson, David Lindsay. *Scientists Are Human* (London: Watts, 1938).

Watts, Eric King. "'Voice' and 'Voicelessness' in Rhetorical Studies." *Quarterly Journal of Speech* 87 (2001) 179–96.

Weaver, Richard M. *The Ethics of Rhetoric.* 1953. Reprint, Davis, CA: Hermagoras Press, 1985.

Weijer, Charles. "The Breast Cancer Research Scandal: Addressing the Issues." *Canadian Medical Association Journal* 152 (1995): 1195–97.

———. "For and Against: Clinical Equipoise and Not the Uncertainty Principle Is the Moral Underpinning of the Randomised Controlled Trial." *British Medical Journal* 321 (2000): 756–58.

Weinberg, Alvin. "Impact of Large-Scale Science on the United States." *Science* 134 (1961): 161–64.

Weiss, Rick. "NIH: The Price of Neglect." *Science* 251, no. 4993 (1991): 508–11.

"What Is Truth?" Editorial. *Lancet* 343, no. 8911 (1994): 1443–44.

Wilmshurst, Peter. "The Code of Silence." *Lancet* 349, no. 9051 (1997): 567–69.

Wilsdon, James, B. Wynne, and J. Stilgoe. *The Public Value of Science; or, How to Ensure That Science Really Matters.* London: Demos, 2005.

Yalom, Marion. *A History of the Breast.* New York: HarperCollins, 1997.

Zagacki, Kenneth S., and William Keith. "Rhetoric, *Topoi*, and Scientific Revolutions." *Philosophy and Rhetoric* 25, no. 1 (1992): 59–78.

Zeneca Pharmaceuticals. "Heroes Among Us." *Solutions: Business News and Commentary for Zeneca Pharmaceuticals U.S. Employees* 2, no. 3 (1998). Copy on file with the author.

Zerbe, Michael, Amanda J. Young, and Edwin R. Nagelhout. "The Rhetoric of Fraud in Breast Cancer Trials: Manifestations in Medical Journals and the Mass Media—And Missed Opportunities." *Journal of Technical Writing and Communication* 28 (1998): 39–61.

Ziman, John. *An Introduction to Science Studies: The Philosophical and Social Aspects of Science and Technology.* New York: Cambridge University Press, 1984.

Zones, Jane S. "Profits from Pain: The Political Economy of Breast Cancer." In Kasper and Ferguson, *Breast Cancer,* 119–51.

Zuckerman, Harriet. "Deviant Behavior and Social Control in Science." In *Deviance and Social Change,* edited by E. Sagarin, 87–138. Beverly Hills, CA: Sage, 1977.

Index